Psychology of Emotions, Motivations and Actions

Expression and Control of the Pain Body

PSYCHOLOGY OF EMOTIONS, MOTIVATIONS AND ACTIONS

Additional books in this series can be found on Nova's website under the Series tab.

Additional E-books in this series can be found on Nova's website under the E-books tab.

PAIN AND ITS ORIGINS, DIAGNOSIS AND TREATMENTS

Additional books in this series can be found on Nova's website under the Series tab.

Additional E-books in this series can be found on Nova's website under the E-books tab.

PSYCHOLOGY OF EMOTIONS, MOTIVATIONS AND ACTIONS

EXPRESSION AND CONTROL OF THE PAIN BODY

FERENC MARGITICS

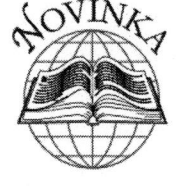

Nova Science Publishers, Inc.
New York

Copyright © 2011 by Nova Science Publishers, Inc.

All rights reserved. No part of this book may be reproduced, stored in a retrieval system or transmitted in any form or by any means: electronic, electrostatic, magnetic, tape, mechanical photocopying, recording or otherwise without the written permission of the Publisher.

For permission to use material from this book please contact us:
Telephone 631-231-7269; Fax 631-231-8175
Web Site: http://www.novapublishers.com

NOTICE TO THE READER

The Publisher has taken reasonable care in the preparation of this book, but makes no expressed or implied warranty of any kind and assumes no responsibility for any errors or omissions. No liability is assumed for incidental or consequential damages in connection with or arising out of information contained in this book. The Publisher shall not be liable for any special, consequential, or exemplary damages resulting, in whole or in part, from the readers' use of, or reliance upon, this material.

Independent verification should be sought for any data, advice or recommendations contained in this book. In addition, no responsibility is assumed by the publisher for any injury and/or damage to persons or property arising from any methods, products, instructions, ideas or otherwise contained in this publication.

This publication is designed to provide accurate and authoritative information with regard to the subject matter covered herein. It is sold with the clear understanding that the Publisher is not engaged in rendering legal or any other professional services. If legal or any other expert assistance is required, the services of a competent person should be sought. FROM A DECLARATION OF PARTICIPANTS JOINTLY ADOPTED BY A COMMITTEE OF THE AMERICAN BAR ASSOCIATION AND A COMMITTEE OF PUBLISHERS.

Additional color graphics may be available in the e-book version of this book.

LIBRARY OF CONGRESS CATALOGING-IN-PUBLICATION DATA
Margitics, Ferenc.
Expression and control of the pain body / Ferenc Margitics.
p. cm.
Includes index.
ISBN 978-1-61728-550-9 (softcover)
1. Pain--Psychological aspects. I. Title.
BF515.M276 2009
152.1'824--dc22
2010022737

Published by Nova Science Publishers, Inc. † New York

Contents

Preface		vii
Chapter 1	Emotions and Pain Body	1
Chapter 2	Psychometric Characteristics of the Pain Body Expression Scale	9
Chapter 3	Psychometric Characteristics of the Pain Body Control Scale	15
Chapter 4	Methodology	19
Chapter 5	Research of the Pain Body	23
Chapter 6	Pain Body and the New Spiritual Consciousness	29
Chapter 7	Pain Body and the Differential Emotions	43
Chapter 8	New Spiritual Consciousness and the Differential Emotions	55
Chapter 9	Pain Body and the Anger Expression	63
Chapter 10	New Spiritual Consciousness and the Anger Expression	71
Chapter 11	Pain Body Expression Scale	77
Chapter 12	Use of the Pain Body Expression Scale	79
Chapter 13	Pain Body Control Scale	81
Chapter 14	Use of the Pain Body Control Scale	83
References		85
Index		89

PREFACE

In Eckhart Tolle's [1, 2] opinion, emotion is the body's reaction to a certain idea, to the mental interpretation of a specific or imaginary situation.

The ideas generating emotional reactions are often pre-verbal, that is, they remain unspoken or even unconscious, and they often appear in early childhood. These unconscious assumptions generate emotions in the body, and these emotions will in turn generate further thoughts or actions.

A negative emotion is one that is poisonous for the body; it upturns the balance and harmonic functions of the body. The carrier of the negative emotions within the individual is the Pain Body.

By "Pain Body," Eckhart Tolle means the emotional pain. Apprehension, hatred, self-pity, remorse, rage, depression, and envyness, etc. are all manifestations of the Pain Body.

All emotional pains suffered by the individual during their life, remain a part of the unconscious of the individual for the rest of their life. All negative emotions, emotional suffering that the individual refuses to face, leave a mark in their unconscious. It is particularly difficult to face with, and to treat, powerful negative emotions in childhood. Such unprocessed emotional pains constitute the foundations of Pain Body.

The author examined the Pain Body with the means of academic psychological research. Following the teachings of Eckhart Tolle, the author formulated a Pain Body Expression Scale (PBES), and a Pain Body Control Scale (PBCS), and carried out their statistical analysis. The purpose has been to develop measuring instruments that may serve as an aid in the recognition of the manifestation of the Pain Body, and also shows the degree of control over the Pain Body.

In the course of his research, the author also wished to find an answer to the question whether a Pain Body as such exists at all, what manifestations it may have, and to what an extent they may be kept under control. The author also examined the connections between the manifestation of the Pain Body and the control over it.

Similarly, any connection between the manifestation and control of the Pain Body and the fundamental emotions of the personality (Interest, Enjoyment, Surprise, Distress, Anger, Disgust, Contempt, Fear, Shame, and Guilt) and the forms of expression of anger (Anger-out, Anger-in), was a subject of research.

A further objective of the research project has been to reveal any possible interrelation between the manifestation and control of Pain Body and the New Spiritual Consciousness and is specific components (Ego-dyastole, Alert consciousness in the present, Transcending the functions of Ego).

ABOUT THE AUTHOR

Dr. Ferenc Margitics, Ph.D. is an Associate Professor and leader of the Health Psychology group at the College of Nyíregyháza, in Hungary. He can be reached at: margif@nyf.hu.

Chapter 1

EMOTIONS AND PAIN BODY

1.1. FUNCTION OF EMOTIONS

The definition of the concept of emotion is one of the most important issues in psychology. Kleinginna and Kleinginna [3] collected the then known 92 definitions of emotion used in psychology in their essay published in 1981. They offered an integrated definition for emotion, based upon the collected previous versions of definition. In their opinion, emotions are complicated clusters of subjective and objective factors, and they are relayed by neurological and hormonal systems.

According to Fischer et al.'s [4] emotion definition, emotions may best be described as a result of a systematic interplay of a number of factors. The following phenomena are included in the emergence of emotions:

- Cognitive procedures (cognitive assessment);
- Patterned physiological processes;
- Willingness for action;
- Subjective feelings;
- Instrumental behavior.

They do not believe that a universal description, equally applicable to all forms of emotion, exists.

Emotions have a wide range of important functions in human life [5, 6]:

- They trigger adaptive reactions preparing the body for external stimuli (e. g. for a fight in the case of a threat);

- They are the primary sources of motivation. They motivate as they call a child's attention to various sources of information in the environment; they energize and prepare the individual to give an adequate answer to external stimuli coming from the environment;
- They play an important role in communication; they have a signaling function and they carry information; (they signal to other people how the individual will react in the situation concerned);
- They reinforce and regulate social relations;
- They exert an influence on cognitive processes (they promote and support processes of perception, memory, and learning)
- Emotions play a prominent role in the regulation of behavior;
- They are instrumental in selecting a behavior that is the best for the individual in a specific situation;
- They play a role in maintaining a specific behavior, in persistence and achieving an objective.

Emotions are therefore extremely important in shaping, keeping together and regulating human relationships.

1.2. Fundamental Emotions

Human emotions cover an extremely wide scale, and it is possible to categorize them according to various aspects.

There are basic human emotions, based upon inherited factors. Such emotions are distinguishable in every culture. These emotions are characterized by a specific structure in the central nervous system, a well discernible vegetative neurological activation pattern, typical mimics and a clearly identifiable quality of experience. These are termed primary basic emotions, because they appear very early in the life of the individual and the facial expressions attached to them are universally recognizable.

Izard [7], in her theory of emotions, describes ten primary basic emotions, which have evolutional adaptive functions. These are the following:

- Interest: the emotional reflection of the neurological activity triggered by novelty. This is the most commonly experienced positive emotion, at the same time a motivational basis of learning, competence, creativity and self-realization. Individuals in the state of interest show attention and curiosity.

- Enjoyment: arises after a creative process; it is the pleasure experienced by the individual after successfully completing an action. Enjoyment is coupled with a sense of self-confidence and the acceptance of the environment. It is not a continually sustainable state.
- Surprise: it is always a transitory state. Surprise or astonishment with its negative counterpart, scare, is the reflection of a powerful neurological reaction caused by a sudden or unexpected event. The biological function of surprise or scare is to discharge the actual emotional state, thus preparing the nervous system for being able to give an adequate response to an unexpected event.
- Distress is the most common negative emotion. It is an emotional state generated by imaginary or real failures and losses. In the case of a series of such experience, it may become a lastingly present emotion.
- Anger: an emotional state triggered by the individual's failure at satisfying a need or accomplishing a purposeful activity. Anger is characterized by rapid energy mobilization and a powerful determination. It is an emotion that protects the integrity and increases the efficiency of the individual.
- Disgust: an emotion generated by physical or psychological decay, urging the individual to escape the circumstances generating the disgust in some way (avoidance or active interference).
- Contempt: from an evolutional aspect, it is a sense of superiority, with the purpose of preparing the individual to face hostile actions. In any situation in which the individual finds it necessary to feel stronger, more intelligent and more civilized than others, superiority and contempt are always there in the background.
- Fear: a negative emotional state, generated by real or imaginary threat. It is usually accompanied by a sense of uncertainty and a sense of being lost.
- Shame/shyness: a negative emotion caused by a sense of social disadvantage. When it is obvious for an individual that for some reason they are unable to meet some kind of a social expectation, they experience shame.
- Guilt: an emotion caused by actions done at the expense or to the disadvantage of others, failure to meet promises made to others, or underperformance in general. Guilt is also experienced when the

individual believes that they have failed to achieve their goals or have not made full use of various opportunities.

Izard [8] verified the clear identifiability of the ten basic emotions through intercultural comparative examinations. As part of the tests, respondents coming from different cultures looked at the pictures of individuals experiencing the emotions concerned. Respondents belonging to various cultural backgrounds unmistakably identified the basic emotions in an identical way.

Genetic heritage, learning and socialization make individuals different in terms of their characteristic combinations or constellations of basic emotions, that is, what combinations of emotions become relatively stable in their lives [9].

Despite the universal nature of the basic emotions, they do not appear in the same way at every individual. The individual expression of emotions is largely influenced by the characteristic features of the cultural background in which the individual grows up.

Another group of emotions is constituted by a higher level of cognitive emotions. Unlike the basic emotions, these are not innate, but they are still universally present. Cognitive processes, e. g. a cognitive evaluation of a specific situation, play an important role in the emergence of these emotions. At these emotions there tends to be much larger cultural differences than those we find at the basic emotions, but a common feature with them is that they also survived because they help in solving the problems posed by an increasingly complex social environment [6].

1.3. Emotional Intelligence

Academic research into emotional intelligence started in the early 1990s. In the period from 1990 to 1993, the concept of emotional intelligence emerged. Mayer and Salovey [10] in their study titled "Emotional intelligence" summarized a large part of the research previously accomplished and, by combining the various research trends, created the formal–skill-based–theory of emotional intelligence and an adequate relevant empirical measuring method.

In the years from 1993 to 1997, the concept of emotional intelligence became popular worldwide, and a series of research programs began [11, 12].

The present period of research into emotional intelligence started in 1998. In this period, the definition of emotional intelligence has been refined and elaborated, and new measuring methods have been developed.

Researchers started exploration at a number of new fields in connection with emotional intelligence. These include–among others–the influence of emotions on social thinking and behavior [13]. The connections between emotional intelligence, alexitimia, maladaptive coping [14], self-actualization [15], marriage [16], empathic punctuality [17], and education [18] is documented.The first definitions of emotional intelligence, referring to skills, were formulated by Mayer et al. in the early 1990s [19]. In their opinion, emotional intelligence was a form of emotional information processing that included an accurate assessment of the emotions of ourselves and of others, the adequate expression of the emotions and an adaptive regulation of the emotions that improved the quality of life.

A few years later, Mayer et al. [20], further developing and expanding their original idea, defined emotional intelligence as the ability of the individual to recognize the significance and connections if emotions, to think and to solve problems as a result. In their opinion, emotional intelligence has a role in the perception of emotions, in the assimilation of feelings attached to the emotions and in the comprehension and management of the emotions.

The characteristic-based definitions of emotional intelligence–as opposed to the skill-based definitions–describe emotional intelligence as a component of abilities or characteristic features.

The characteristic-based models of emotional intelligence are largely different from the skill-based models. Representatives of characteristic-based models use the concept of emotional intelligence as a list of characteristic features or skills through which the individual can be successful in life.

Goleman [12] asserts that emotional intelligence has five components: knowing emotions, managing emotions, self-motivation, recognition of the emotions of others, and managing human relationships. In this approach the emphasis is shifted from the general processing of emotional information, and the skills required for processing, to motivation (here: self-motivation) and to human relationships in general, including the ways in which these relationships are managed.

Bar-On [11] defines emotional intelligence as a complexity of non-cognitive skills, competences and abilities that influence the ability of the individual to cope with the requirements and pressure of the external environment, thus meeting the challenges and expectations posed by daily life.

The Bar-On [11, 21] model contains the five key components of emotional intelligence:

- The ability to recognize, understand and express our emotions and feelings,
- The ability to understand the emotions of others and to establish contact with them,
- The ability to manage and control our emotions,
- The ability to manage changes, process and solve personal and interpersonal problems, and
- The ability to generate positive emotions and the capability of self-motivation.

Each of the five components of emotional intelligence contains a certain number of emotional, personal and social skills and abilities and he facilitators of these skills. The abilities determining behavior intelligent from an emotional and social aspect are the following [11, 21]:

- Self-regard: the ability to understand, accept and respect ourselves,
- Assertiveness: the ability to express emotions, beliefs and ideas and to implement them in a non-destructive way,
- Self-awareness: the ability to recognize and understand emotions,
- Stress-tolerance: the ability of the individual to resist unpleasant events and stressful situations without "falling apart" through an active and positive coping with stress,
- Impulse-control: the ability to resist or delay impulses, drives or calls for action,
- Adaptability: the ability to estimate, compare and evaluate objective and subjectively perceived realities,
- Flexibility: the ability to adapt in emotions, ideas and behavior to changing situations and conditions,
- Problem solving: the ability to identify, interpret and effectively solve problems,
- Empathy: understanding and respecting the feelings of others, and
- Interpersonal relationship: the ability to establish and maintain mutually beneficial interpersonal relationships, characterized by an emotional proximity and a balance in providing and receiving emotions.

The behavior intelligent from emotional and social aspects is supported and facilitated by another five factors. These are the following [11, 21]:

- Optimism: the ability to maintain a positive attitude to life, even during periods of disasters and misfortune,
- Self-realization: the potential ability of the individual to realize their skills and capabilities,
- Happiness: the ability of the individual to be satisfied with life, to see the bright side of things, to find pleasure in work, in themselves and others, to be able to enjoy life in general,
- Independence: self-control and self-guidance in thinking and actions, the ability to be emotionally independent of others, and
- Social responsibility: the ability of the individual to be active, constructive, and cooperative in a social group.

In Bar-On's theory [11, 21] mental abilities such as emotional self-awareness is linked with other characteristic features–independent of mental abilities–such as independence and self-esteem or mood. Despite of the wide scope of the model, Bar-On [11, 21] formulated the expectations in connection with it with care and reservation. In his/her opinion, emotional intelligence is a simply and opportunity for achieving success, and not success itself.

1.4. PAIN BODY

In Eckhart Tolle's [1, 2] opinion, emotion is the body's reaction to a certain idea, to the mental interpretation of a specific or imaginary situation.

The ideas generating emotional reactions are often pre-verbal, that is, they remain unspoken or even unconscious, and they often appear in early childhood. These unconscious assumptions generate emotions in the body, and these emotions will in turn generate further thoughts or actions.

A negative emotion is one that is poisonous for the body, it upturns the balance and harmonic functions of the body. The carrier of the negative emotions within the individual is the Pain Body.

By "Pain Body," Eckhart Tolle [1, 2] means the emotional pain. Apprehension, hatred, self-pity, remorse, rage, depression, envy, etc. are all manifestations of the Pain Body.

All emotional pains suffered by the individual during their life, remain a part of the unconscious of the individual for the rest of their life. All negative emotions, and emotional suffering that the individual refuses to face leave a mark in their unconscious. It is particularly difficult to face with, and to treat, powerful negative emotions in childhood. Such unprocessed emotional pains constitute the foundations of Pain Body.

In the collective unconscious, every individual carries their own share of collective human pain that also belongs to the Pain Body.

The emotional component of the Ego is constituted by the unprocessed emotions concentrated in the Pain Body. They occupy human mind. Pain is inseparable from the Ego state identified with the mind.

Ego means the conventional, ordinary "self," which constitutes the common mistake in which the illusory belief in the personal identity is rooted. This illusory self will then be the basis of all mental processes, human relations and the interpretation of reality. The structure of the ego is an unconscious factor, which forces the individual to reinforce his/her identity by joining an external object. The content of the ego will then be the thing with which the individual indentified him/herself (my house, my car, my child, my intelligence, my opinion, etc.).

The emotional components of Ego are different in every individual; they are larger in some people and smaller in others.

At most people, Pain Body has a dormant and an active state. Events that coincide with patterns of pain previously experienced by the individual may easily activate Pain Body. An apparently insignificant event may active an old pain in the individual, retrieving thoughts and emotions caused by old pains that occurred several years previously. Physical or emotional abuse, loss, a sense of abandonment may activate Pain Body particularly easily.

Any enjoyment, emotionally high state also hides the potential of pain in it, and this pain may with time be manifested. Enjoyment may therefore be transformed into some form of pain.

Chapter 2

PSYCHOMETRIC CHARACTERISTICS OF THE PAIN BODY EXPRESSION SCALE

As the first step in the compilation of the questionnaire, we defined the construction (Pain Body Expression) that we intended to measure with the scale. For an operational definition of the construction, we formulated statements, following the teachings of Eckhart Tolle [1, 2].

This primary scale, consisting of 25 statements (scale: 1= virtually never, 2=sometimes, 3= frequently, 4=almost always), was tested with the help of 300 individuals (150 men, 150 women).

The criteria for selecting the appropriate items were the following:

- ➢ Selecting the items characterized by the largest item-surplus correlation;
- ➢ The items should be clearcut, easily identifiable ones, thus eliminating items containing redundant elements.

When the scale was finalized, only the most reliable statements were retained, and the ones not matching the criteria above were omitted. In this way, the final number of items was 17.

For the item-surplus correlations, the average values for each items and the dispersion see Chart 1.

The item surplus correlations express the relationship of the items with the totality of the remainder items.

The reliability of the final version of the scale is indicated by the high value of the inner consistency (Cronbach-alfa=0,89). The indicators of internal consistency were similar at both genders.

Chart 1. The item-surplus correlations and descriptive statistical figures of the Pain Body Expression Scale

Item of Pain Body Expression Scale	Item-Remainder correlation	Mean Value	Standard Deviation
1. I become upset without any particular reason	0,64	1,64	0,62
2. I harbor resentment against others	0,61	1,96	0,65
3. I easily become angry	0,62	2,19	0,71
4. I feel remorse	0,57	2,21	0,69
5. My moods change rapidly	0,58	2,28	0,90
6. I become depressed or sad without any particular reason	0,51	1,75	0,77
7. People make me nervous	0,56	1,80	0,69
8. I am overcome by self-pity	0,57	1,53	0,65
9. I am often overcome by my emotions	0,61	2,50	0,82
10. I have negative ideas about myself	0,49	2,02	0,79
11. I am envious of others	0,54	1,54	0,61
12. I easily offend others	0,57	1,85	0,83
13. Small, insignificant things trigger intensive emotions in me	0,50	2,52	0,81
14. I easily criticize others	0,51	2,23	0,90
15. I am often overcome by my emotions unexpectedly	0,52	2,09	0,85
16. I am unhappy	0,61	1,73	0,67
17. I am impatient with others	0,59	2,1	0,83

The reliability of the scale and its particular items for an extended period of time was tested with the help of a group of 140 college students (70 women and 70 men). The reliability of the scale was found to be good again (Chart 2).

Chart 2. Indicators of the reliability of the Pain Body Expression Scale over an extended period of time

Item of Pain Body Expression Scale	Test-retest (n=140)
1. I become upset without any particular reason	0,86
2. I harbour resentment against others	0,79
3. I easily become angry	0,81
4. I feel remorse	0,82
5. My moods change rapidly	0,89
6. I become depressed or sad without any particular reason	0,80
7. People make me nervous	0,78
8. I am overcome by self-pity	0,77
9. I am often overcome by my emotions	0,81
10. I have negative ideas about myself	0,82
11. I am envious of others	0,86
12. I easily offend others	0,89
13. Small, insignificant things trigger intensive emotions in me	0,81
14. I easily criticize others	0,84
15. I am often overcome by my emotions unexpectedly	0,79
16. I am unhappy	0,87
17. I am impatient with others	0,85

The strength of the interrelations was indicated by the Kaiser-Meyer-Olkin (KMO) value. The KMO value was in our case 0,698, which indicates the applicability of the variables for a factor analysis.

As a result of the factor analysis, the statements on the scale were arranged into three factors, explaining 68,2% of the variance.

The first factor (eigenvalue: 4,506) explained 28,7 per cent of the complete variance. The following items of the Pain Body Expression Scale belonged to this factor:

The factor structure of the questionnaire was also examined, with the results summed up in Chart 3.

The criterion of the applicability of the factor analysis is that the data items should be in interrelation with each other, and the variables should contain redundant information.

Chart 3. The factor structure of the Pain Body Expression Scale

Item of Pain Body Expression Scale	Factors		
	1	2	3
I become upset without any particular reason	0,548		
I easily become angry	0,511		
My moods change rapidly	0,440		
People make me nervous	0,637		
I easily offend others	0,553		
I easily criticize others	0,837		
I am impatient with others	0,565		
I harbour resentment against others		0,459	
I feel remorse		0,673	
I have negative ideas about myself		0,690	
I am envious of others		0,693	
I am unhappy		0,507	
I become depressed or sad without any particular reason			0,528
I am overcome by self-pity			0,562
I am often overcome by my emotions			0,763
Small, insignificant things trigger intensive emotions in me			0,660
I am often overcome by my emotions unexpectedly			0,508

- I become upset without any particular reason
- I easily become angry
- My moods change rapidly
- People make me nervous
- I easily offend others
- I easily criticize others
- I am impatient with others

This factor comprises impatience, exasperation, nervousness and the criticism and offence directed to other people, so this factor is named *"Exasperation" sub-scale.*

The second factor (eigenvalue: 2.876) explained 23.3 per cent of the total variance. The following items of the Pain Body Expression Scale belonged to this factor:

- I harbor resentment against others
- I feel remorse
- I have negative ideas about myself
- I am envious of others
- I am unhappy

This factor comprises grudge, unhappiness, and guilt individuals direct towards themselves and other people, so this factor is named *"Grudge" sub-scale.*

The third factor (eigenvalue: 2.102) explained the 16,2 per cent of the total variance. The following items of the New Spiritual Consciousness Scale belonged to this factor:

- I become depressed or sad without any particular reason
- I am overcome by self-pity
- I am often overcome by my emotions
- Small, insignificant things trigger intensive emotions in me
- I am often overcome by my emotions unexpectedly

This factor shows the dynamics of the emergence of emotions, so we named this *sub-scale "Inflamability"*

Chapter 3

PSYCHOMETRIC CHARACTERISTICS OF THE PAIN BODY CONTROL SCALE

As the first step in the compilation of the questionnaire, we defined the construction (Pain Body Control) that we intended to measure with the scale. For an operational definition of the construction, we formulated statements, following the teachings of Eckhart Tolle [1, 2].

This primary scale, consisting of 15 statements (scale: 1= virtually never, 2=sometimes, 3= frequently, 4=almost always), was tested with the help of 300 individuals (150 men, 150 women).

The criteria for selecting the appropriate items were the following:

- ➤ Selecting the items characterized by the largest item-surplus correlation;
- ➤ The items should be clearcut, easily identifiable ones, thus eliminating items containing redundant elements.

When the scale was finalized, only the most reliable statements were retained, and the ones not matching the criteria above were omitted. In this way, the final number of items was 7.

For the item-surplus correlations, the average values for each items and the dispersion see Chart 4.

The item surplus correlations express the relationship of the items with the totality of the remainder items.

The reliability of the final version of the scale is indicated by the high value of the inner consistency (Cronbach-alfa=0,85). The indicators of internal consistency were similar at both genders.

Chart 4. The item-surplus correlations and descriptive statistical figures of the Pain Body Control Scale

Item of Pain Body Control Scale	Item-Remainder correlation	Mean Value	Standard Deviation
1. I am able to control my emotions	0,53	2,54	0,89
2. I am able to forget about old offenses	0,56	2,50	0,88
3. When I realize that an emotions overcomes me, I am able to consciously suppress it	0,47	2,59	0,83
4. I am able to contemplate my emotions like an outsider	0,41	2,08	0,85
5. I do not identify with my emotions, I simply allow them to happen	0,48	1,86	0,92
6. When I am suffering emotionally, I do not escape, I make efforts to consciously face the emotion concerned	0,51	2,98	0,86
7. I am able to focus my attention on the present, instead of re-living old emotions	0,49	2,54	0,87

Chart 5. Indicators of the reliability of the Pain Body Control Scale over an extended period of time

Item of Pain Body Control Scale	Test-retest (n=140)
1. I am able to control my emotions	0,81
2. I am able to forget about old offenses	0,78
3. When I realize that an emotions overcomes me, I am able to consciously suppress it	0,72
4. I am able to contemplate my emotions like an outsider	0,74
5. I do not identify with my emotions, I simply allow them to happen	0,81
6. When I am suffering emotionally, I do not escape, I make efforts to consciously face the emotion concerned	0,86
7. I am able to focus my attention on the present, instead of re-living old emotions	0,88

Chart 6. The factor structure of the Pain Body Control Scale

Item of Pain Body Expression Scale	Factor
	1
1. I am able to control my emotions	0,509
2. I am able to forget about old offenses	0,617
3. When I realize that an emotions overcomes me, I am able to consciously suppress it	0,817
4. I am able to contemplate my emotions like an outsider	0,791
5. I do not identify with my emotions, I simply allow them to happen	0,454
6. When I am suffering emotionally, I do not escape, I make efforts to consciously face the emotion concerned	0,646
7. I am able to focus my attention on the present, instead of re-living old emotions	0,579

The reliability of the scale and its particular items for an extended period of time was tested with the help of a group of 140 college students (70 women and 70 men). The reliability of the scale was found to be good again (Chart 5).

The factor structure of the questionnaire was also examined, with the results summed up in Chart 6.

The criterion of the applicability of the factor analysis is that the data items should be in interrelation with each other, and the variables should contain redundant information. The strength of the interrelations was indicated by the Kaiser- Meyer- Olkin (KMO) value. The KMO value was in our case 0,809, which indicates the applicability of the variables for a factor analysis.

As a result of the factor analysis, the statements on the scale were arranged into three factors, explaining 74,8% of the variance.

Chapter 4

METHODOLOGY

4.1. PARTICIPANTS

We measured the pravelence of Pain Body Expression Scale and Pain Body Control Scale among college students.

Data was collected among students at the College of Nyíregyháza. We collected data randomly at every faculty and participation was voluntary and it was done with their consent. 500 students took part in the research and 484 of them provided valuable data (302 women and 182 men).

The average age was 20,77 (standard deviation 1.71) the median value was 21 years

4.2. MEASURES

The following research methods were used:

4.2.1. Examination of Expression of the Pain Body

To study examination of Pain Body, we applied the Pain Body Expression Scale.

4.2.2. Examination of Control of the Pain Body

To study control of Pain Body, we applied the Pain Body Control Scale.

4.2.3. Examination of the New Spiritual Consciousness

To study New Spiritual Consciousness, we applied the New Spiritual Consciousness Scale [22].

Margitics [22] developed the New Spiritual Consciousness Scale for the New Spiritual Consciousness test. The inventory is suitable for the examination of certain dimensions of New Spiritual Consciousness.

The questionnaire describes the following dimensions of New Spiritual Consciousness:

- Ego-Dyastole (reduction in the functions of Ego)
- Alert Consciousness in the Present
- Transcending the Functions of Ego

With the help of a frequency scale it examines how often the specific dimensions of New Spiritual Consciousness appear. Participants in the examination will enter the frequency into a six-grade scale (1=never or almost never, 2= rarely, 3=sometimes, 4= on the majority of days, 5= every day, and 6= many times a day)

4.2.4. Examination of the Differential Emotions

To study examination of Differential Emotions, we applied the Hungarian version of Differential Emotions Scale [7].

Izard [7] developed Differential Emotions Scale in order to differentiate between the basic emotions. The inventory is suitable for examining the ability of experiencing certain basic emotions as a permanent characteristic feature.

With the help of a frequency scale it examines how often the basic emotions appear. Participants in the examination will enter the frequency into a four-grade scale (1=virtually never, 2=sometimes, 3=frequently, 4=almost always).

Differential Emotions Scale consists of a scale identifying ten basic emotions. The questionnaire describes the following fundamental emotions:

- Trait of Interest
- Trait of Enjoyment
- Trait of Surprise
- Trait of Distress

- Trait of Anger
- Trait of Disgust
- Trait of Contempt
- Trait of Fear
- Trait of Shame
- Trait of Guilt
- Trait of Anxiety

The Hungarian adaptation of the questionnaire was done by Oláh [7], who found the reliability of the scales good (Cronbach-alpha=0,49-0,76).

4.2.5. Examination of the Anger Expression

To study examination of Anger Expression, we applied the Hungarian version of Anger Expression Scale [7].

Anger Expression Scale was compiled by Spielberger et al [23] in order to measure the open expression or suppression of anger and wrath as a permanent characteristic feature. The scale shows how often the individual examined experiences the emotion of anger and wrath and how they express the emotion of anger: whether they show it in an aggressive way, pouring it on their partners, or they suppress and control it (experiencing anger without open aggression.)

With the help of a frequency scale it examines how often the anger appears. Participants in the examination will enter the frequency into a four-grade scale (1=virtually never, 2=sometimes, 3=frequently, and 4=almost always).

The questionnaire describes the following dimensions of Anger Expression:

- Anger Expression
- Anger in
- Anger out

The Hungarian adaptation of the questionnaire was done by Oláh [7], who found the reliability of the scales good (Cronbach-alpha=0,76).

Chapter 5

RESEARCH OF THE PAIN BODY

5.1. RESEARCH OF THE PAIN BODY EXPRESSION

The descriptive and comparative statistics of the findings achieved with Pain Body Expression Scale is provided (for the whole of the sample and in a breakdown according to the two genders) in Chart 7.

Chart 7. The descriptive and comparative statistics of the Pain Body Expression Scale

	Total (n=484)		Women (n=302)		Men (n=182)	
	Mean Value	Standard Deviation	Mean Value	Standard Deviation	Mean Value	Standard Deviation
Pain Body Expression Scale	34,1	6,7	34,6	7,7	33,7	6,3

The chart clearly shows that, according to the scores on the Pain Body Expression Scale, there is no considerable difference between men and women

Figure 1 contains the descripritive statistics of the results of subscales of the Pain Body Expression. In order to make the figures comparative, the average values and dispersions are set to one answer on the scale.

An examination of the composition of Pain Body indicates that while women are characterized by Inflammability, men are primarily characterized by Grudge.

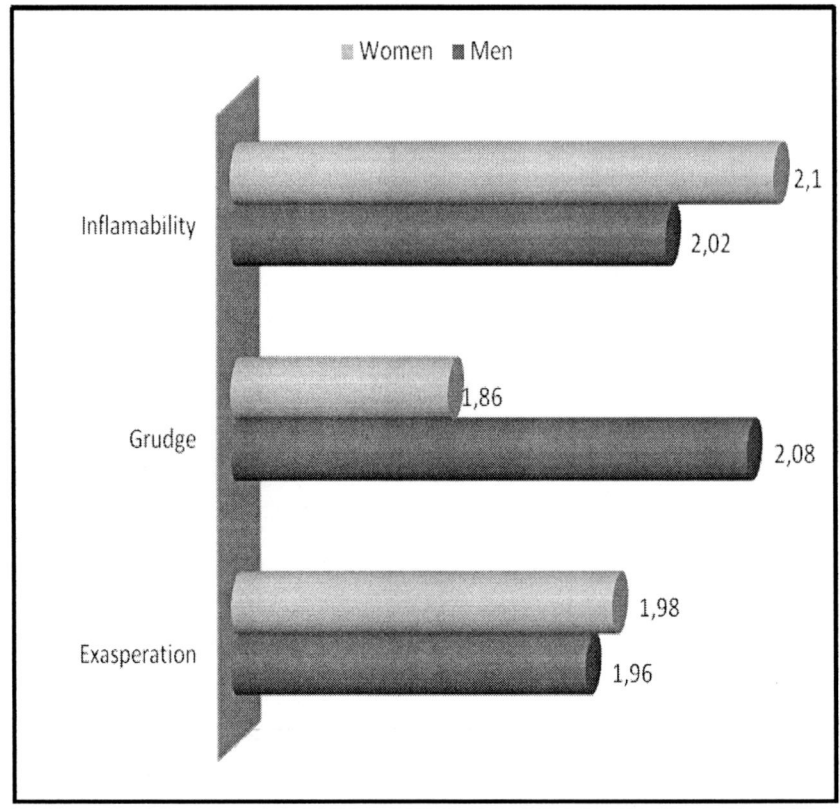

Figure 1. The descriptive statistics of subscales of the Pain Body Expression.

As far as the components of Pain Body are concerned, the second most powerful factor in the case of the women was Exasperation, in the case of the men it was Inflammability. The weakest component was Grudge in the case of the women and Exasperation in the case of the men. The differences above were, however, not very large, and did not reach a significant level according to the results of the comparative statistical analysis.

5.2. RESEARCH OF THE PAIN BODY CONTROL

The descriptive and comparative statistics of the findings achieved with Pain Body Control Scale is provided (for the whole of the sample and in a breakdown according to the two genders) in Chart 8.

Chart 8. The descriptive and comparative statistics of the Pain Body Control Scale

	Total (n=484)		Women (n=302)		Men (n=182)	
	Mean Value	Standard Deviation	Mean Value	Standard Deviation	Mean Value	Standard Deviation
Pain Body Control Scale	17,3	3,9	16,7	3,9	18,5	3,9

The chart suggests that, according to the results achieved on the Pain Body Control Scale, men tend to have a somewhat more powerful emotional control than women.

According to the results of the comparative statistical analysis, the difference between the two genders is not significant.

5.3. INTERRELATION BETWEEN PAIN BODY CONTROL WITH THE PAIN BODY EXPRESSION

Chart 9 contains the connection of certain dimensions of subscales of the Pain Body Expression with the Pain Body Control Scale (Pearson correlation) for the whole sample and for men and women separately.

Chart 9. The connection of certain dimensions of subscales of the Pain Body Expression with the Pain Body Control Scale (Pearson correlation)

	Exasperation Subscale	Grudge Subscale	Inflamability Subscale	Pain Body Expression Scale
Total (n=484)				
Pain Body Control Scale	-0,195	-0,028	-0,254*	-0,246*
Women (n=302)				
Pain Body Control Scale	-0,232*	-0,118	-0,271*	-0,290**
Men (n=182)				
Pain Body Control Scale	-0,034	-0,088	-0,231*	-0,224*

** Correlation is significant at the 0.01 level.
* Correlation is significant at the 0.05 level.

At the entire sample, there was a close, significant negative correlation between Pain Body Control and Pain Body, which was found to be even more powerful in the case of the women than in the case of the men. It means that emotional control may be more powerful when Pain Body is weaker.

At the entire sample, Inflammability was the item on the Pain Body Expression sub-scale that was found to be in a close, significant negative correlation with Pain Body Control. In this respect, there was no considerable difference between the two genders. It means that emotional control is more powerful and effective at a less inflammable Pain Body.

In the case of the women, Pain Body Control was also found to be in a close, significant negative correlation with Exasperation. It suggests that, in the case of the women, emotional control is more powerful and effective when the Pain Body is less susceptible for exasperation.

Our research did not reveal any close correlation between Grudge sub-scale and Pain Body Control.

5.4. Discussion

In the course of our research project we did not find any difference between the two genders in terms of the evolution of the Pain Body. We identified three components of the Pain Body, which have different qualities and different functions. The three components are the following:

- ➢ Exasperation (impatience, nervousness, anxiety, criticizing and offending other people)
- ➢ Grudge (grudge directed against himself/herself and other people, unhappiness and guilt)
- ➢ Inflammability (the dynamics of the emergence of emotions)

All the three components of the Pain Body were identified at both sexes, and no considerable structural differences were found at the two genders

No considerable difference between the two genders was found in terms of the control of Pain Body either.

When examining the interrelation between Pain Body Control and Pain Body, we found that the individuals with a powerless Pain Body tend to have a more powerful emotional control.

As for the specific components of Pain Body this interrelation was observed particularly at the lower levels of Inflammability and Exasperation, and not at Grudge.

Emotional control is more powerful in the presence of weaker Inflammability and Exasperation, but it does not apply to a powerless Grudge.

Chapter 6

PAIN BODY AND THE NEW SPIRITUAL CONSCIOUSNESS

6.1. PAIN BODY EXPRESSION AND THE NEW SPIRITUAL CONSCIOUSNESS

For the composition of the examination groups, the results scored on the Pain Body Expression Scale.

Students were arranged according to their position of the Pain Body Expression Scale. Students low on the Pain Body Expression Scale were in the first quarter (powerless Pain Body), whereas those who were high on the scale were put in the fourth quarter (powerful Pain Body) (Chart 10).

The group of powerless Pain Body created according to the Pain Body Expression Scale consisted of 131 individuals (85 women, 46 men), that with a powerful Pain Body consisted of 122 people (79 women and 43 men).

Figure 2 contains the descripritive statistics (mean value) of the results of New Spiritual Consciousness Scale, employed in the groups arranged according to the Pain Body Expression Scale.

Chart 10. The quartiles of Pain Body Expression Scale

	Quartiles	
	first	fourth
Pain Body Expression Scale	>30	38<

The results indicate that, regardless of gender, individuals with a powerless Pain Body are characterized by New Spiritual Consciousness to a significantly higher degree than individuals with a powerful Pain Body (Total: t=3,882, p<0,000; Women: t=3,282, p<0,002; Men: t=3,354, p<0,000).

The correlation between the sub-scales of New Spiritual Consciousness and Pain Body was also examined.

Figure 3 contains the descripritive statistics (mean value) of the results of "Ego-Dyastole" Subscale, employed in the groups arranged according to the Pain Body Expression Scale.

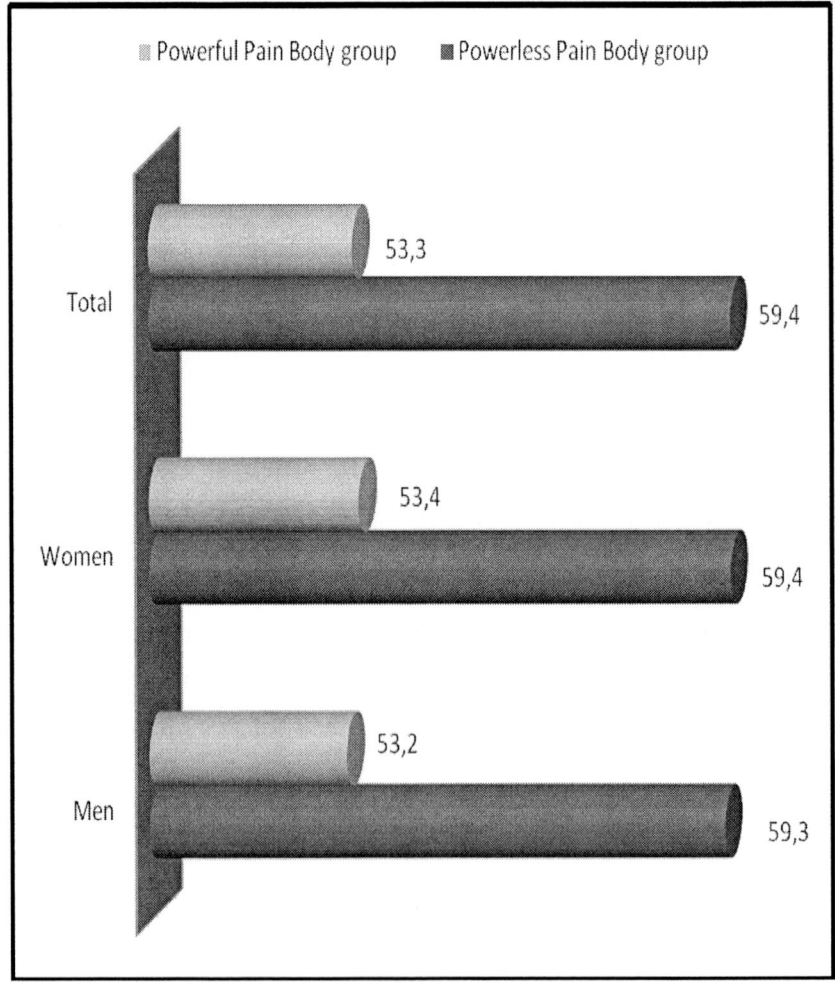

Figure 2. Descriptive statistics (mean value) of the results of New Spiritual Consciousness Scale, employed in the groups arranged according to the Pain Body Expression Scale.

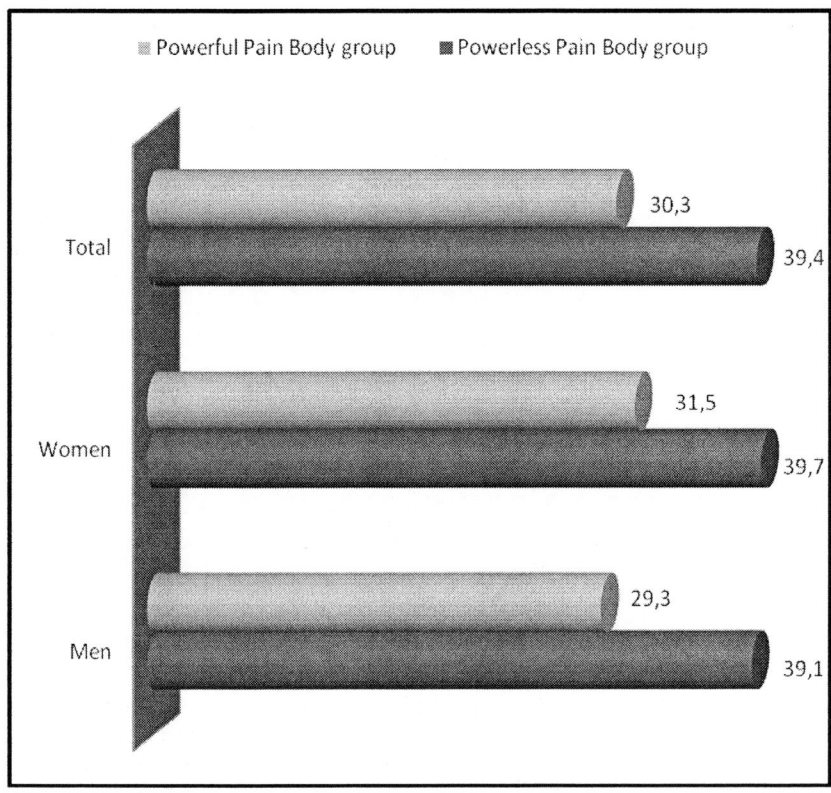

Figure 3. Descriptive statistics (mean value) of the results of "Ego-Dyastole" Subscale, employed in the groups arranged according to the Pain Body Expression Scale.

As indicated by our findings, people with a powerless Pain Body, regardless of gender, are characterized by a tendency of the functions of the Ego to decline to a larger extent than people with a powerful Pain Body are (Total: t=8,749, p<0,000; Women: t=6,987, p<0,000; Men: t=7,426, p<0,000)

Figure 4 contains the descripritive statistics (mean value) of the results ofAlert Consciousness in the Present" Subscale, employed in the groups arranged according to the Pain Body Expression Scale.

Our findings suggest that people with a powerful Pain Body, regardless of gender, are characterized by the presence of alert consciousness in the present to a larger extent than individuals with a powerful Pain Body are (Total: t=2,243, p<0,029; Women: t=2,221, p<0,032; Men: t=2,238, p<0,021)

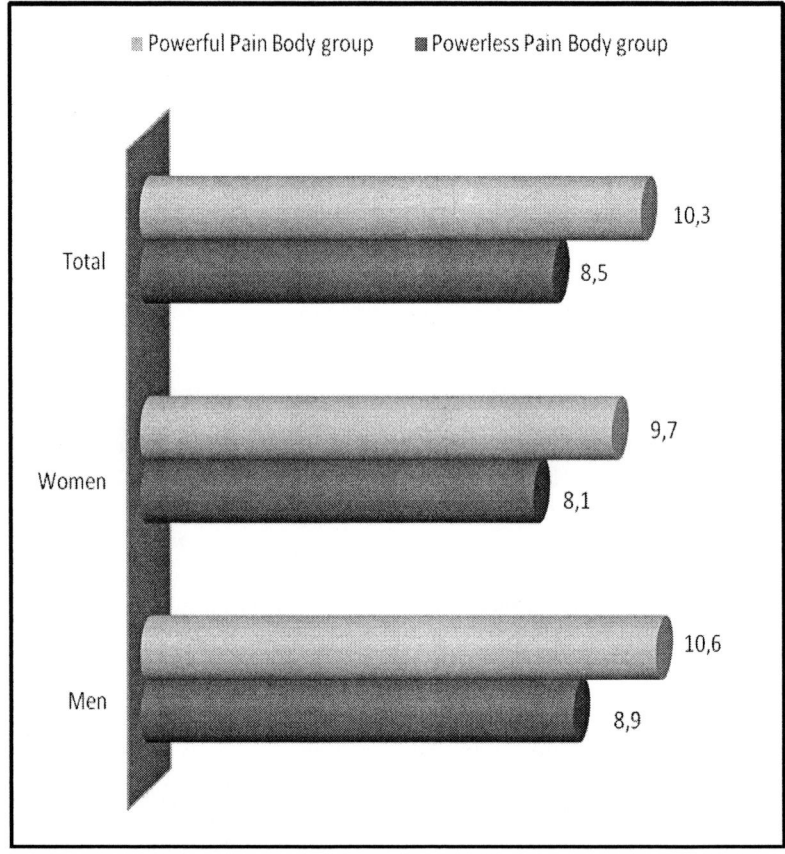

Figure 4. Descriptive statistics (mean value) of the results of "A lert Consciousness in the Present" Subscale, employed in the groups arranged according to the Pain Body Expression Scale.

Figure 5 contains the descripritive statistics (mean value) of the results of "Transcending the Functions of Ego" Subscale, employed in the groups arranged according to the Pain Body Expression Scale.

It is shown in the figure that individuals with a powerful Pain Body, regardless of gender, are more capable of overcoming the functions of the Ego than individuals with a powerless Pain Body. The difference between the two groups was, however, not significant.

In the following part of the survey, we carried out a linear regression analysis (stepwise method) for the whole of the sample and for each gender separately to analyse the various dimensions of New Spiritual Consciousness.

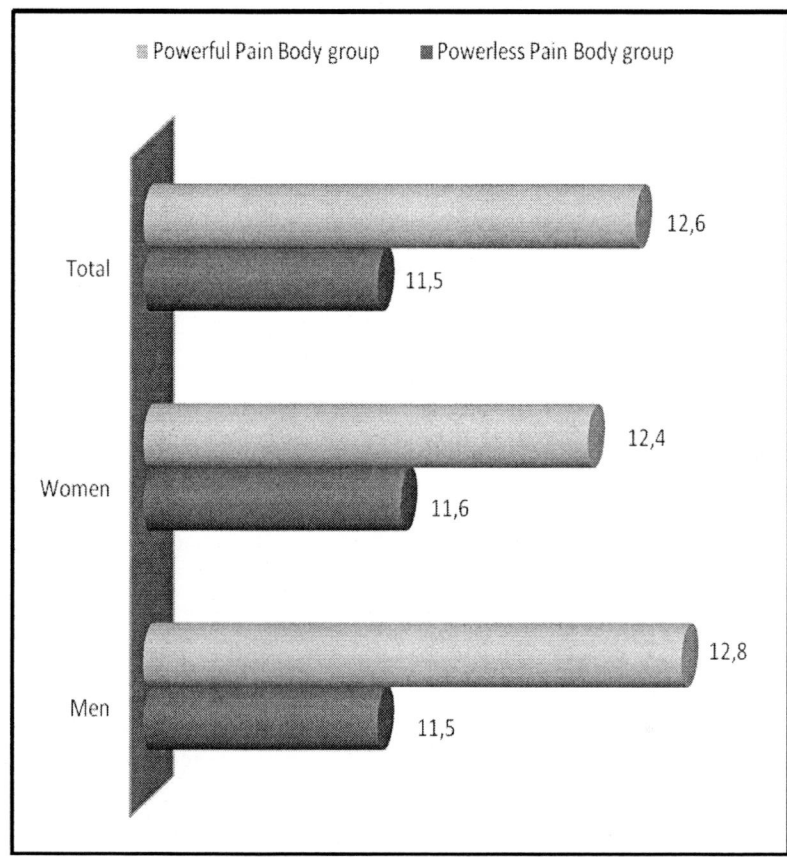

Figure 5. Descriptive statistics (mean value) of the results of "Transcending the Functions of Ego" Subscale, employed in the groups arranged according to the Pain Body Expression Scale.

In the examination, the results achieved on the Pain Body Expression Scale were the dependent variables and the various dimensions of New Spiritual Consciousness were the predictors (Chart 11).

At the entire sample, Pain Body was only found to be in a close, significant negative correlation with Ego-Dyastole of all the dimensions of New Spiritual Consciousness, explaining 49,7% of the variance of the Pain Body.

An examination of the two genders separately revealed that the tendency was the same in the case of both sexes, explaining 41,3% of the variance of the PB in the case of the women and 53,4% in the case of the men.

Chart 11. The regression of the results scored on the Pain Body Expression Scale on the various sub-scales measuring New Spiritual Consciousness (approved models; p<0,05)

Predictor	Béta	t	p<
Total: $F_{totál}=92,789$; $df=1/484$; $p<0,000$			
"Ego-dyastole" sub-scale	-0,705	-9,633	0,000
Women: $F_{totál}=52,166$; $df=1/302$; $p<0,000$			
"Ego-dyastole" sub-scale	-0,634	-7,223	0,000
Men: $F_{totál}=51,465$; $df=1/182$; $p<0,000$			
"Ego-dyastole" sub-scale	-0,761	-7,716	0,000

Chart 12. The regression of the results scored on the "Exasperation" Subscale on the various sub-scales measuring New Spiritual Consciousness (approved models; p<0,05)

Predictor	Béta	t	p<
Total: $F_{totál}=41,841$; $df=1/484$; $p<0,000$			
"Ego-dyastole" sub-scale	-0,555	-6,468	0,000
Women: $F_{totál}=10,906$; $df=1/302$; $p<0,000$			
"Ego-dyastole" sub-scale	-0,542	-5,555	0,000
Men: $F_{totál}=17,235$; $df=1/182$; $p<0,000$			
"Ego-dyastole" sub-scale	-0,699	-7,149	0,000

It means that there is a direct proportion between the increase of the power of the Pain Body and the structure and content of Ego.

The structure of the Ego is an unconscious factor, which forces the individual to reinforce his/her identity by joining an external object. The content of the ego will then be the thing with which the individual indentified him/herself (my house, my car, my child, my intelligence, my opinion etc.).

In the examination, the results achieved on the "Exasperation" Subscale were the dependent variables and the various dimensions of New Spiritual Consciousness were the predictors (Chart 12).

At the entire sample, Pain Body was only found to be in a close, significant negative correlation with Exasperation of all the dimensions of New Spiritual Consciousness, explaining 30,8%, of the variance of the Pain Body.

Chart 13. The regression of the results scored on the "Grudge" Subscale on the various sub-scales measuring New Spiritual Consciousness (approved models; p<0,05)

Predictor	Béta	t	p<
Total: $F_{totál}=24,338$; $df=1/484$; $p<0,000$			
Ego-dyastole" sub-scale	-0,567	-6,737	0,000
"Transcending the Functions of Ego" subscale	-0,181	-2,156	0,034
Women: $F_{totál}=14,175$; $df=1/302$; $p<0,000$			
Ego-dyastole" sub-scale	-0,434	-4,366	0,000
"Transcending the Functions of Ego" subscale	-0,304	-3,060	0,003
Men: $F_{totál}=30,403$; $df=1/182$; $p<0,000$			
"Ego-dyastole" sub-scale	-0,687	-7,514	0,000

An examination of the two genders separately revealed that the tendency was the same in the case of both sexes, explaining 29,4% of the variance of the PB in the case of the women and 37,8% in the case of the men.

It suggests that there is a direct proportion between the increase of Exasperation and the structure and content of Ego at the individual concerned.

In the examination, the results achieved on the "Grudge" Subscale were the dependent variables and the various dimensions of New Spiritual Consciousness were the predictors (Chart 13).

At the entire sample, Grudge was only found to be in a close, significant negative correlation with Ego-dyastole of all the dimensions of New Spiritual Consciousness, explaining 34,4% of the variance of the Pain Body.

An examination of the two genders separately revealed that the tendency was the same in the case of the women, explaining 28% of the variance of the Pain Body. In the case of the men, Grudge only showed a significant close negative relationship with the Ego-dyastole, explaining 42,3% of the variance.

In the examination, the results achieved on the "Inflammability" Subscale were the dependent variables and the various dimensions of New Spiritual Consciousness were the predictors (Chart 14).

At the entire sample, Pain Body was only found to be in a close, significant negative correlation with Inflammability of all the dimensions of

New Spiritual Consciousness, explaining 25,6%, of the variance of the Pain Body.

Chart 14. The regression of the results scored on the "Inflamability" Subscale on the various sub-scales measuring New Spiritual Consciousness (approved models; p<0,05)

Predictor	Béta	t	p<
Total: $F_{totál}=32,380; df=1/484; p<0,000$			
"Ego-dyastole" sub-scale	-0,506	-5,690	0,000
Women: $F_{totál}=19,858; df=1/302; p<0,000$			
"Ego-dyastole" sub-scale	-0,460	-4,456	0,000
Men: $F_{totál}=18,011; df=1/182; p<0,000$			
"Ego-dyastole" sub-scale	-0,614	-4,244	0,000

An examination of the two genders separately revealed that the tendency was the same in the case of both sexes, explaining 21,2% of the variance of the Pain Body in the case of the women and 34,3% in the case of the men.

6.2. PAIN BODY CONTROL AND THE NEW SPIRITUAL CONSCIOUSNESS

For the composition of the examination groups, the results scored on the Pain Body Control Scale.

Students were arranged according to their position of the Pain Body Control Scale. Students low on the Pain Body Control Scale were in the first quarter (powerless control), whereas those who were high on the scale were put in the fourth quarter (powerful control) (Chart 15).

Chart 15. The quartiles of Pain Body Control Scale

	Quartiles	
	first	fourth
Pain Body Control Scale	>14	20<

The group of powerless control created according to the Pain Body Control Scale consisted of 128 individuals (88 women, 40 men), that with a powerful control consisted of 125 people (76 women and 49 men).

Figure 6 contains the descriptive statistics (mean value) of the results of New Spiritual Consciousness Scale, employed in the groups arranged according to the Pain Body Control Scale.

The results indicate that, regardless of gender, individuals with a powerful Pain Body Control are characterized by New Spiritual Consciousness to a significantly higher degree than individuals with a powerless Pain Body Control. (Total: t=4,359, p<0,000; Women: t=4,050, p<0,000; Men: t=4,521, p<0,000)

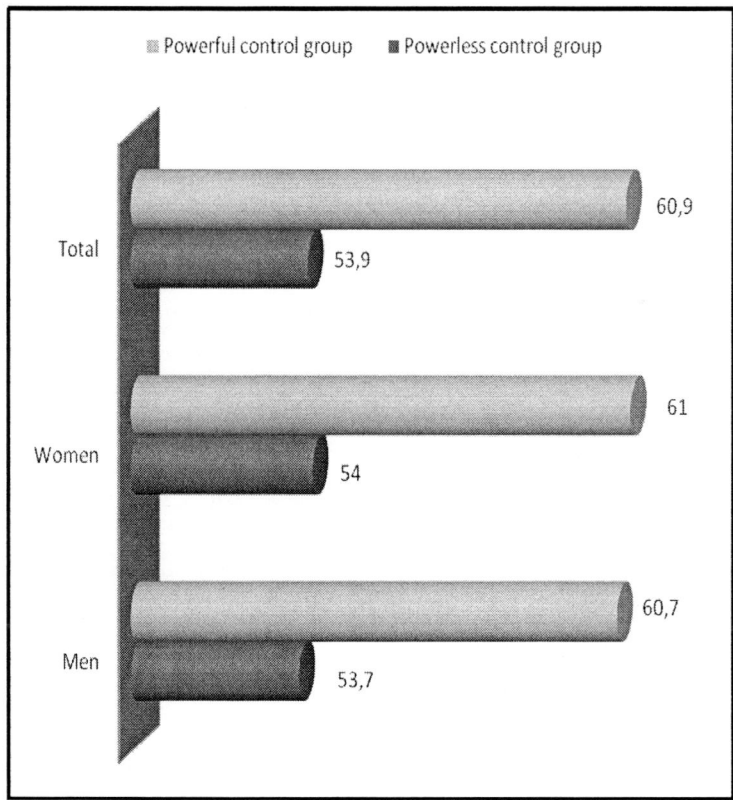

Figure 6. Descriptive statistics (mean value) of the results of New Spiritual Consciousness Scale, employed in the groups arranged according to the Pain Body Control Scale.

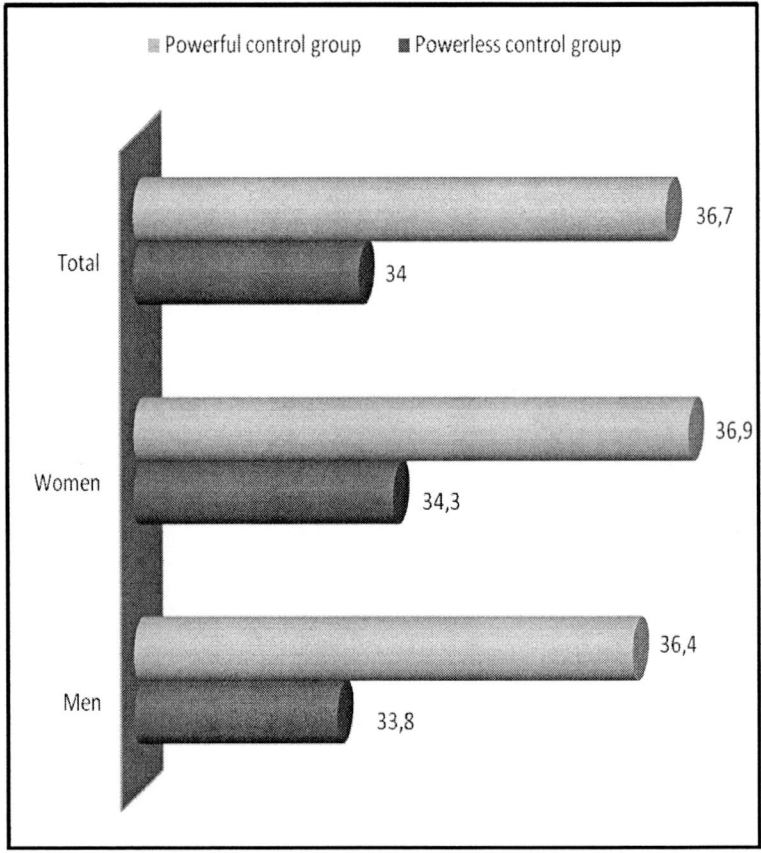

Figure 7. Descriptive statistics (mean value) of the results of "Ego-Dyastole" Subscale, employed in the groups arranged according to the Pain Body Control Scale.

We also wished to examine the interrelations between the specific subscales of New Spiritual Consciousness and emotional control.

Figure 7 contains the descriptive statistics (mean value) of the results of "Ego-Dyastole" Subscale, employed in the groups arranged according to the Pain Body Control Scale.

Our findings suggest that individuals with a powerful emotional control, regardless of gender, are characterized by the decline of the functions of the Ego to a larger extent than individuals with a powerless control. The difference between the two groups was, however, not significant.

Figure 8 contains the descriptive statistics (mean value) of the results of "Alert Consciousness in the Present" Subscale, employed in the groups arranged according to the Pain Body Control Scale.

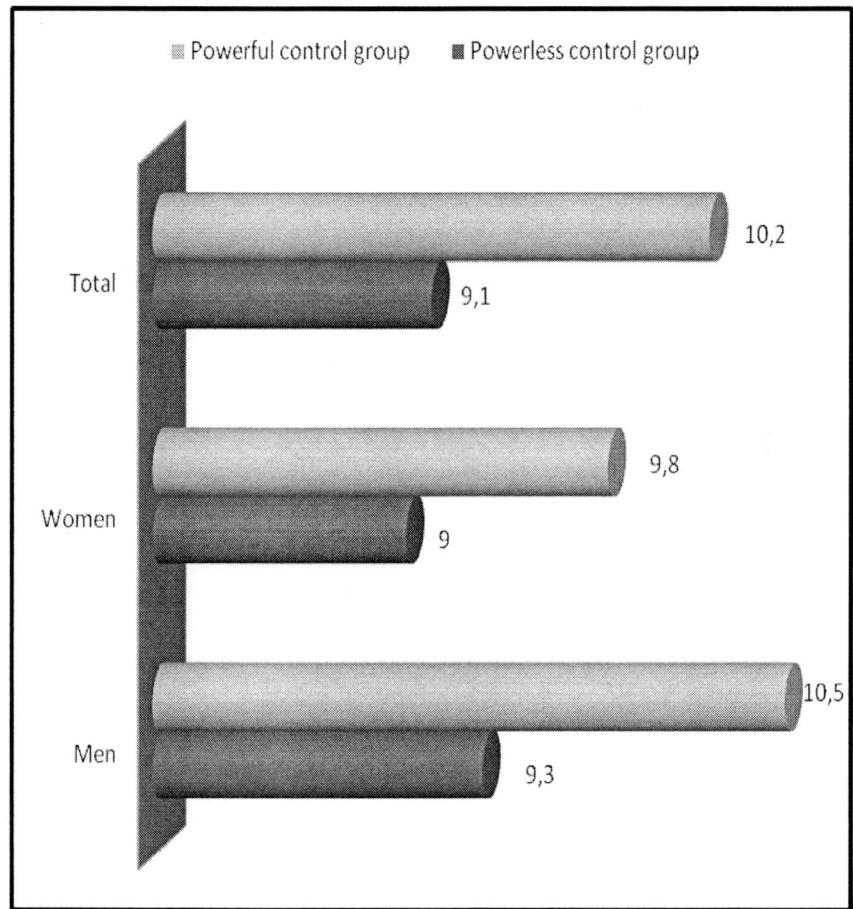

Figure 8. Descriptive statistics (mean value) of the results of "Alert Consciousness in the Present" Subscale, employed in the groups arranged according to the Pain Body Control Scale.

Our results indicate that individuals with a powerful emotional control, regardless of gender, are characterized by alert consciousness in the present to a larger extent than individuals with a powerless control. The difference between the two groups was, however, not significant.

Figure 9 contains the descripritive statistics (mean value) of the results of Transcending the Functions of Ego" Subscale, employed in the groups arranged according to the Pain Body Control Scale.

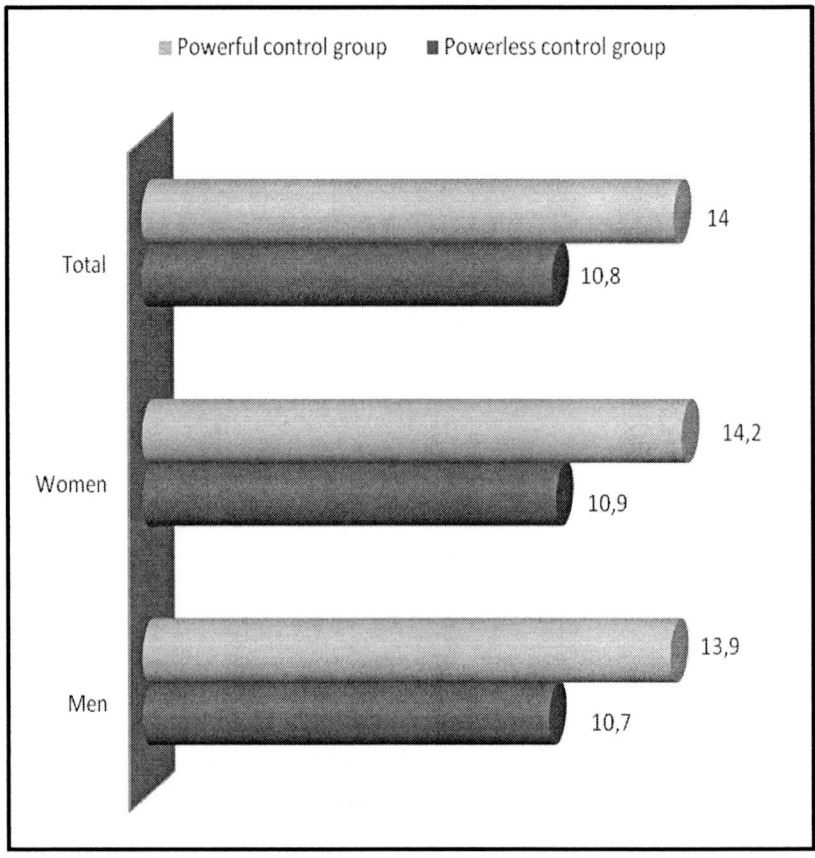

Figure 9. Descriptive statistics (mean value) of the results of "Transcending the Functions of Ego" Subscale, employed in the groups arranged according to the Pain Body Control Scale.

The figure indicates that individuals with a powerful emotional control, regardless of gender, were characterized by a significantly higher degree of ability to overcome the functions of the Ego than the individuals with powerless control (Total: t=3,294, p<0,002; Women: t=3,183, p<0,003; Men: t=3,138, p<0,002).

In the following part of the survey, we carried out a linear regression analysis (stepwise method) for the whole of the sample and for each gender separately to analyse the various dimensions of New Spiritual Consciousness.

Chart 16. The regression of the results scored on the Pain Body Control Scale on the various sub-scales measuring New Spiritual Consciousness (approved models; p<0,05)

Predictor	Béta	t	p<
Total: Ftotál=8,324; df=1/484; p<0,005			
"Transcending the Functions of Ego" subscale	0,285	2,885	0,005
Women: Ftotál= 7,996; df=1/302; p<0,006			
"Transcending the Functions of Ego" subscale	0,312	2,828	0,006
Men: Ftotál= 6,152; df=1/182; p<0,023			
"Transcending the Functions of Ego" subscale	0,294	2,481	0,023

In the examination, the results achieved on the Pain Body Control Scale were the dependent variables and the various dimensions of New Spiritual Consciousness were the predictors (Chart 16).

At the entire sample, emotional control was only found to be a close, significant positive correlation with the Transcending the Functions of Ego of all the dimensions of New Spiritual Consciousness, explaining 27,2% of the variance.

An examination of the two genders separately revealed that the tendency was the same at both sexes, explaining 31,2% of the variance of the emotional control at the women and 25,8% at the men.

It means that there is a direct proportion between the increase of the level of emotional control and the increase of the level of the ability of overcoming the functions of the Ego at the individuals participating in the survey.

6.3. DISCUSSION

In Eckhart Tolle's [1, 2] interpretation, our present consciousness opens up the gate to spirituality. The individual must experience the present moment, while the alertness of his/her consciousness enables the person to view his or her own thoughts, emotions and reactions triggered by the stimuli of the environment.

The Presence thus created (conscious alertness) brings about the sense of tranquility and internal peace. The sustained conscious attention launches the spiritual process of transubstantiation that leads the individual to a new spiritual consciousness, new perspective and new ways of observations.

An emerging Presence alters the individual's relationship to their own Pain Body.

In the course of our research project we examined what relationship links Pain Body and Pain Body Control to Presence-that is, the New Spiritual Consciousness expressing it and its specific dimensions.

Our findings indicate that, regardless of gender, the only specific component of New Spiritual Consciousness that had a close connection with Pain Body was Ego-Dyastole. It means that in the case of a powerless Pain Body the structure and content of the Ego are also powerless and the other way around. This interrelation was observed at all the structural components of Pain Body.

On the other hand, we found that individuals with a powerful Pain Body were characterized by an alert consciousness in the presence to a larger extent than individuals with a powerless Pain Body. This was the case with both genders. It is possible that this interrelation is not powered by Pain Body, but by some other factors, which are not discussed as part of this research project.

An examination of the interrelations between Pain Body Control and New Spiritual Consciousness - regardless of gender- revealed that Transcending the Functions of Ego was the only dimension of New Spiritual Consciousness which was in a close connection with Pain Body Control the New Spiritual Consciousness. It means that there is a direct proportion between the increase of the power of Pain Body Control and the increase of the individual's willingness to overcome the functions of the Ego.

Individuals with a powerful Pain Body Control were characterized by a decline of the functions of the Ego and the alert consciousness in the present to a larger extent than individuals with a powerless control. This tendency was the same at both genders. The interrelation may, however, not be based upon the extent of Pain Body Control but on some other factor not subject of this research.

Chapter 7

PAIN BODY AND THE DIFFERENTIAL EMOTIONS

7.1. PAIN BODY EXPRESSION AND THE DIFFERENTIONAL EMOTIONS

For the composition of the examination groups, the results scored on the Pain Body Expression Scale.

Students were arranged according to their position of the Pain Body Expression Scale. Students low on the Pain Body Expression Scale were in the first quarter (powerless Pain Body), whereas those who were high on the scale were put in the fourth quarter (powerful Pain Body).

Figure 10. contains the descriptive statistics (mean value) of the results of Differential Emotions Scale, employed in the groups arranged according to the Pain Body Expression Scale.

The figure indicates that individuals with a powerful Pain Body, regardless of gender, have a richer variety of ways of expressing their emotions than the individuals with powerless control. The difference was found to be significant at both genders (Total: $t=5,659$, $p<0,000$; Women: $t=5,894$, $p<0,000$; Men: $t=5,452$, $p<0,000$)

Figure 11. contains the descripritive statistics (mean value) of the results of emotions of Differential Emotions Scale, employed in the groups arranged according to the Pain Body Expression Scale.

The figure suggests that the individuals possessing a powerful Pain Body also possess more powerful traits of emotions than the individuals having a powerless Pain Body.

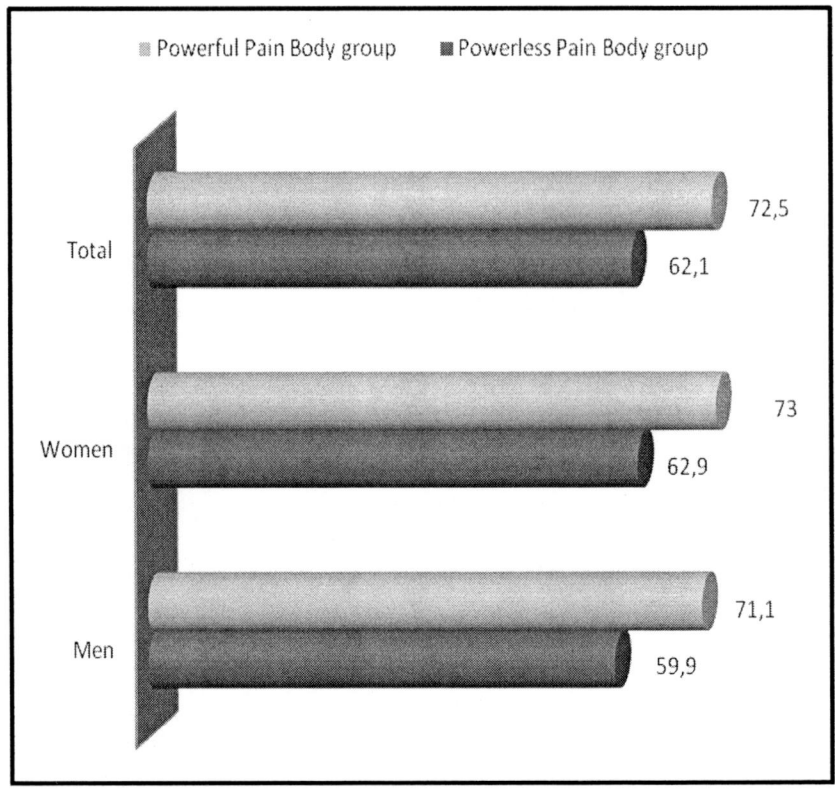

Figure 10. Descriptive statistics (mean value) of the results of Differentional Emotions Scale, employed in the groups arranged according to the Pain Body Expression Scale.

The differences between the two groups only reached a significant level at the following traits:

- Trait of Enjoyment (t=2,733, p<0,008)
- Trait of Distress (t=5,120, p<0,000)
- Trait of Anger (t=5,048, p<0,000)
- Trait of Disgust (t=5,151, p<0,000)
- Trait of Contempt (t=2,636, p<0,011)
- Trait of Shame (t=3,328, p<0,002)
- Trait of Guilt (t=3,955, p<0,000)
- Trait of Fear (t=2,230, p<0,030)

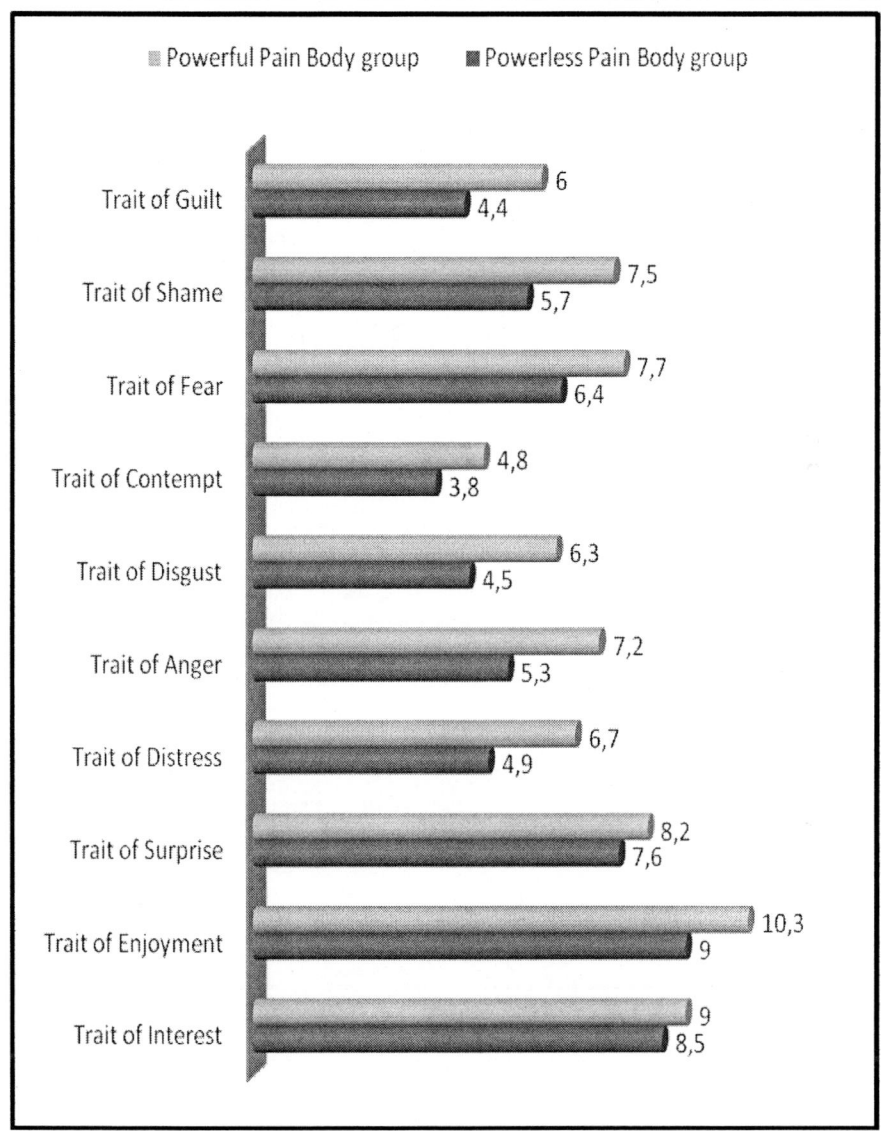

Figure 11. Descriptive statistics (mean value) of the results of emotions of Differentional Emotions Scale, employed in the groups arranged according to the Pain Body Expression Scale.

In the following part of the survey, we carried out a linear regression analysis (stepwise method) for the whole of the sample and for each gender separately to analyze the various sub-scales of Differentional Emotions Scale.

In the examination, the results achieved on the Pain Body Expression Scale were the dependent variables and the various sub-scales of Differential Emotions were the predictors (Chart 17).

At the entire sample, Pain Body was found to be in a significant, close positive correlation with Disgust, Shame and Guilt of all the dimensions of emotion expression, explaining 45% of the variance of the Pain Body.

At the genders separately, the tendency in the case of the men was the same as that at the entire sample, explaining 54,3% of the variance of the Pain Body.

In the case of the women, Pain Body was also in a significant, close positive correlation with the Traits of Disgust and Shame. Anger and Contempt were added to the previous two emotions among those that were in close interrelation with Pain Body at the women. These emotions explained 49,4% of the variance of Pain Body in the case of the women.

It means that there is a direct proportion between the increase of power of Pain Body and the Traits of Disgust, Shame, Anger and Contempt at the women and with Disgust, Shame, Anger and Contempt at the men.

In the examination, the results achieved on the "Exasperation" Subscale were the dependent variables and the various sub-scales of Differential Emotions were the predictors (Chart 18).

Chart 17. The regression of the results scored on the Pain Body Expression Scale on the various sub-scales measuring Differential Emotions (approved models; p<0,05)

Predictor	Béta	t	p<
Total: $F_{totál}=25,050$; $df=1/484$; $p<0,000$			
Trait of Disgust	0,412	4,989	0,000
Trait of Shame	0,351	3,428	0,000
Trait of Guilt	0,163	2,022	0,046
Women: $F_{totál}=17,304$; $df=1/302$; $p<0,000$			
Trait of Disgust	0,389	3,958	0,000
Trait of Shame	0,281	3,276	0,002
Trait of Anger	0,266	2,822	0,006
Trait of Contempt	0,185	2,020	0,047
Men: $F_{totál}=39,094$; $df=1/182$; $p<0,000$			
Trait of Disgust	0,427	4,253	0,000
Trait of Shame	0,372	3,612	0,000
Trait of Guilt	0,187	2,458	0,034

Chart 18. The regression of the results scored on the "Exasperation" Subscale on the various sub-scales measuring Differentional Emotions (approved models; p<0,05

Predictor	Béta	t	p<
Total: $F_{totál}=27,756$; $df=1/484$; $p<0,000$			
Trait of Disgust	0,377	4,185	0,000
Trait of Anger	0,349	3,873	0,000
Women: $F_{totál}= 23,113$; $df=1/302$; $p<0,000$			
Trait of Disgust	0,398	4,072	0,000
Trait of Anger	0,323	3,436	0,001
Trait of Contempt	0,191	2,128	0,037
Men: $F_{totál}= 19,164$; $df=1/182$; $p<0,000$			
Trait of Disgust	0,389	4,378	0,000
Trait of Anger	0,285	3,128	0,002

Chart 19. The regression of the results scored on the Grudge" Subscale on the various sub-scales measuring Differentional Emotions (approved models; p<0,05)

Predictor	Béta	t	p<
Total: $F_{totál}=19,617$; $df=1/484$; $p<0,000$			
Trait of Shame	0,364	4,272	0,000
Trait of Distress	0,298	3,423	0,001
Trait of Guilt	0,222	2,746	0,007
Trait of Contempt	0,165	2,122	0,037
Women: $F_{totál}= 17,989$; $df=1/302$; $p<0,000$			
Trait of Shame	0,447	4,610	0,000
Trait of Distress	0,309	3,225	0,002
Trait of Contempt	0,275	3,053	0,003
Men: $F_{totál}= 17,654$; $df=1/182$; $p<0,000$			
Trait of Shame	0,398	3,684	0,000
Trait of Distress	0,312	3,547	0,000
Trait of Guilt	0,257	2,987	0,005

At the entire sample, Exasperation was found to be in a close, significant positive correlation with Disgust and Distress of all the dimensions of emotion expression, explaining 49,7% of the variance of Exasperation.

At the two genders, the tendency was the same as that observed at the entire sample. In the case of the women it explained 47,4% of the variance of Exasperation, whereas the figure was 51,6% in the case of the men.

It suggests that at both sexes the Traits of Disgust and Anger increase together with the increase of Exasperation, to which a little Contempt is added.

In the examination, the results achieved on the "Grudge" Subscale were the dependent variables and the various sub-scales of Differential Emotions were the predictors (Chart 19).

At the entire sample, Grudge appeared to be in a significant, close positive correlation with the Traits of Shame, Distress, Guilt and Contempt, all these explaining 46,3% of the variance of the Grudge.

At the two genders, the tendency of the Traits of Shame and Distress was the same as that observed at the entire sample. At women, the Trait of Contempt, at men the Trait of Guilt was added. These emotions explained 42,8% of the variance of Grudge at women, whereas the figure was 49,6% in the case of the men. It suggests that at both sexes the Traits of Shame and Distress increase together with the increase of Grudge, to which a little Trait of Contempt is added at women and a similar Trait of Guilt at the men.

In the examination, the results achieved on the "Inflammability" Subscale were the dependent variables and the various sub-scales of Differential Emotions were the predictors (Chart 20).

Chart 20. The regression of the results scored on the "Inflamability" Subscale on the various sub-scales measuring Differentional Emotions (approved models; p<0,05)

Predictor	Béta	t	p<
Total: $F_{totál}=16,981$; $df=1/484$; $p<0,000$			
Trait of Shame	0,326	3,444	0,000
Trait of Disgust	0,304	3,207	0,002
Women: $F_{totál}=8,330$; $df=1/302$; $p<0,000$			
Trait of Shame	0,348	3,291	0,000
Trait of Disgust	0,243	2,296	0,018
Men: $F_{totál}=10,154$; $df=1/182$; $p<0,000$			
Trait of Shame	0,348	3,453	0,000
Trait of Disgust	0,254	2,314	0,015

At the entire sample, Inflammability was found to be in a significant, close positive correlation with the inclination to express Shame and Disgust, all these explaining 26,7% of the variance of the Inflammability.

At the two genders, the tendency was the same as that observed at the entire sample. In the case of the women it explained 25,7% of the variance of Inflammability, whereas the figure was 27,8% in the case of the men.

It suggests that the Traits of Shame and Disgust increase in parallel with the increase of Inflammability.

7.2. PAIN BODY CONTROL AND THE DIFFERENTIONAL EMOTIONS

For the composition of the examination groups, the results scored on the Pain Body Control Scale.

Students were arranged according to their position of the Pain Body Control Scale. Students low on the Pain Body Control Scale were in the first quarter (powerless Control), whereas those who were high on the scale were put in the fourth quarter (powerful Control).

Figure 12 contains the descriptive statistics (mean value) of the results of Differentional Emotions Scale, employed in the groups arranged according to the Pain Body Control Scale.

It is shown in the figure that individuals with a powerless emotional control, regardless of gender, tend to have a more powerful inclination to express their emotions that people with a powerful emotional control. The difference between the two groups, hoever, only reached a significant level in the case of the women ($t=2,158$, $p<0,037$).

Figure 13 contains the descriptive statistics (mean value) of the results of emotions of Differentional Emotions Scale, employed in the groups arranged according to the Pain Body Control Scale.

Individuals with a powerful emotional control were found to be considerably more willing to express the following emotions than individuals with a powerless emotional control:

- Trait of Interest ($t=2,546$, $p<0,014$
- Trait of Enjoyment ($t=2,152$, $p<0,036$)

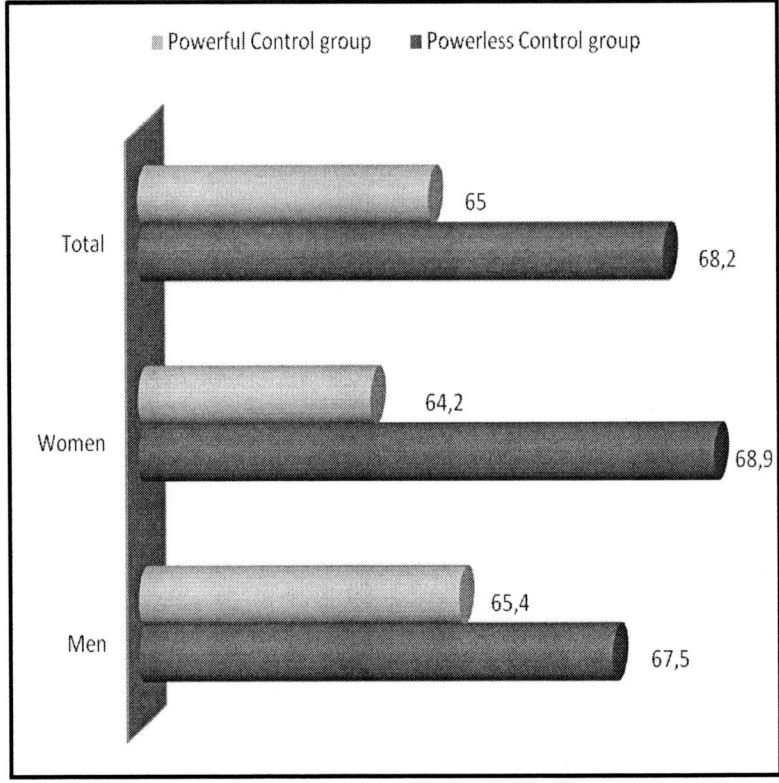

Figure 12. Descriptive statistics (mean value) of the results of Differentional Emotions Scale, employed in the groups arranged according to the Pain Body Control Scale.

Individuals with a powerless emotional control were found to be considerably more willing to express the following emotions than individuals with a powerful emotional control:

> Trait of Distress (t=2,173, p<0,034)
> Trait of Anger (t=2,169, p<0,037)
> Trait of Disgust (t=2,241, p<0,029)
> Trait of Fear (t=2,106, p<0,040)

In terms of other emotions there was no significant difference between the two groups.

In the following part of the survey, we carried out a linear regression analysis (stepwise method) for the whole of the sample and for each gender separately to analyze the various sub-scales of Differentional Emotions Scale.

In the examination, the results achieved on the Pain Body Control Scale were the dependent variables and the various sub-scales of Differential Emotions were the predictors (Chart 21).

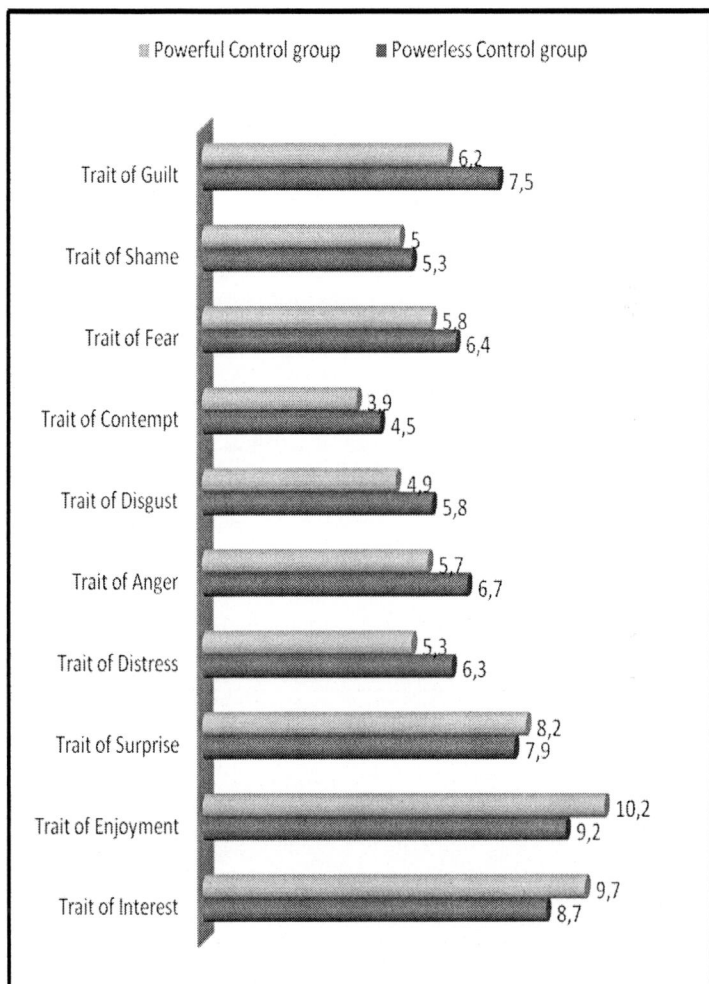

Figure 13. Descriptive statistics (mean value) of the results of emotions of Differential Emotions Scale, employed in the groups arranged according to the Pain Body Control Scale.

Chart 21. The regression of the results scored on the Pain Body Control Scale on the various sub-scales measuring Differential Emotions (approved models; p<0,05)

Predictor	Béta	t	p<
Total: Ftotál=6,672; df=1/484; p<0,011			
Trait of Enjoyment	0,257	2,583	0,011
Women: Ftotál= 10,305; df=1/302; p<0,002			
Trait of Enjoyment	0,350	3,210	0,002
Men: Ftotál= 7,154; df=1/182; p<0,009			
Trait of Enjoyment	0,278	2,876	0,009

At the entire sample, emotional control was only found to be in a significant, close positive relationship with the Trait of Enjoyment only, explaining 6,6% of the variance of emotional control.

At the two genders, the tendency was the same as that observed at the entire sample. In the case of the women it explained 8,2% of the variance of emotional control, whereas the figure was 5,1% in the case of the men.

It means that there is a direct proportion between the increase of emotional control and the Trait of Enjoyment.

7.3. DISCUSSION

Our research was also extended to the interrelation between Pain Body/Pain Body Control and the willingness to express various emotions.

Our findings suggest that Pain Body was in a close connection with the expression of Disgust and Shame at both genders. In addition to that, women were found to be more willing to express Anger and Contempt. It means that there is a direct proportion between the decline of the power of Pain Body and the decline of the willingness to express Disgust, Shame and Anger at women and the willingness to express Disgust and Shame at men and the other way around.

As for the specific components of Pain Body, Exasperation was closely linked to the expression of Disgust and Anger at both sexes. It means that there is a direct proportion between the decline of Exasperation and the decline of the willingness to express Disgust and Shame. In the case of the women, the reduction of the willingness to express Contempt was added to the other two emotions.

Grudge was found to be in a close correlation with the willingness to express Shame and Distress at both genders. At women, the willingness to express Contempt, and at the men the willingness to express Guilt was added to the two emotions the two sexes shared. It means that with the decline of Grudge, the readiness to express Shame and Distress also declines at both sexes. At women, it is coupled with the decline of the willingness to express Contempt, and at the men the willingness to express Guilt declined.

Inflammability appeared to be in a close interrelation with the inclination to express Shame and Disgust at both men and women. It indicates that there is a direct proportion between the decline of Inflammability and the decline of willingness to express Shame and Disgust. The tendency was the same at both sexes.

When examining the connections between Pain Body Control and the expression of emotions we found that, regardless of gender, the emotional control was in a close correlation with the willingness to express Enjoyment only.

It means that there is a direct proportion between the increase of emotional control and the Trait of Enjoyment.

Chapter 8

NEW SPIRITUAL CONSCIOUSNESS AND THE DIFFERENTIAL EMOTIONS

For the composition of the examination groups, the results scored on the New Spiritual Consciousness Scale.

Students were arranged according to their position of the New Spiritual Consciousness Scale. Students low on the New Spiritual Consciousness Scale were in the first quarter, whereas those who were high on the scale were put in the fourth quarter (Chart 22).

Chart 22. The quartiles of New Spiritual Consciousness Scale

	Quartiles	
	first	fourth
New Spiritual Consciousness Scale	>52	62<

The group of low spiritual consciousness created according to the New Spiritual Consciousness Scale consisted of 128 individuals (83 women, 45 men), that with a high spiritual consciosness consisted of 124 people (81women and 43 men).

Figure 14. contains the descripritive statistics (mean value) of the results of Differentional Emotions Scale, employed in the groups arranged according to the New Spiritual Consciousness Scale.

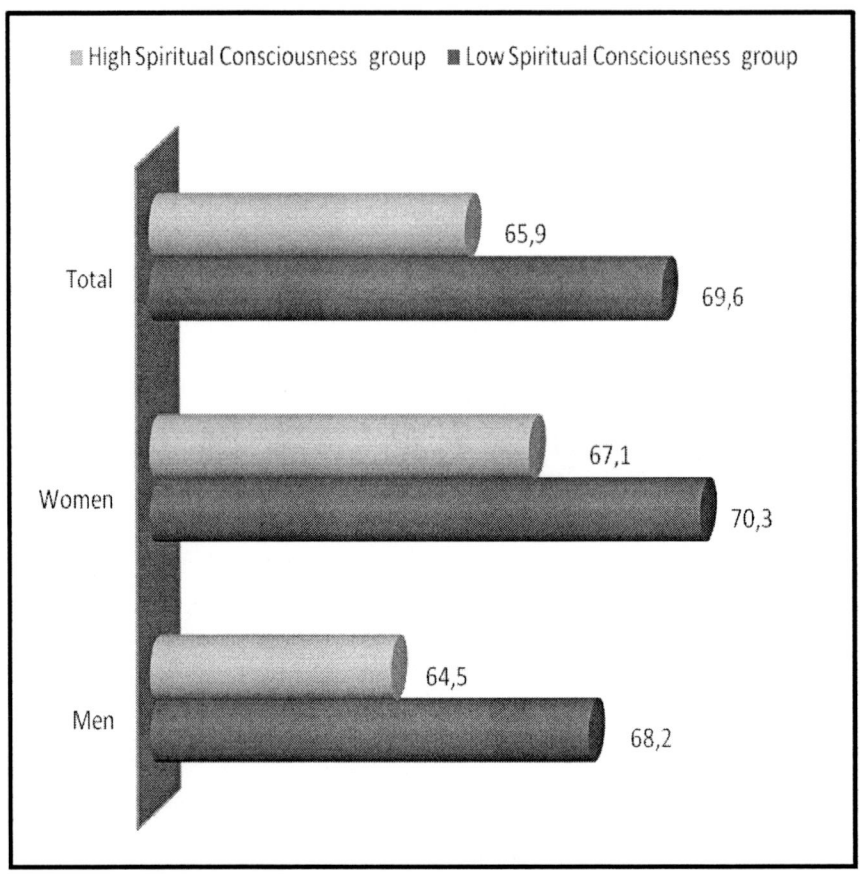

Figure 14. Descriptive statistics (mean value) of the results of Differentional Emotions Scale, employed in the groups arranged according to the New Spiritual Consciousness Scale.

The figure suggests that the individuals characterized by a lower level of new spiritual consciousness tend to show more willingness to express their emotions than the individuals with a higher level of new spiritual consciousness, although the difference between the two groups was not significant at either sex.

Figure 15. contains the descripritive statistics (mean value) of the results of emotions of Differentional Emotions Scale, employed in the groups arranged according to the New Spiritual Consciousness Scale.

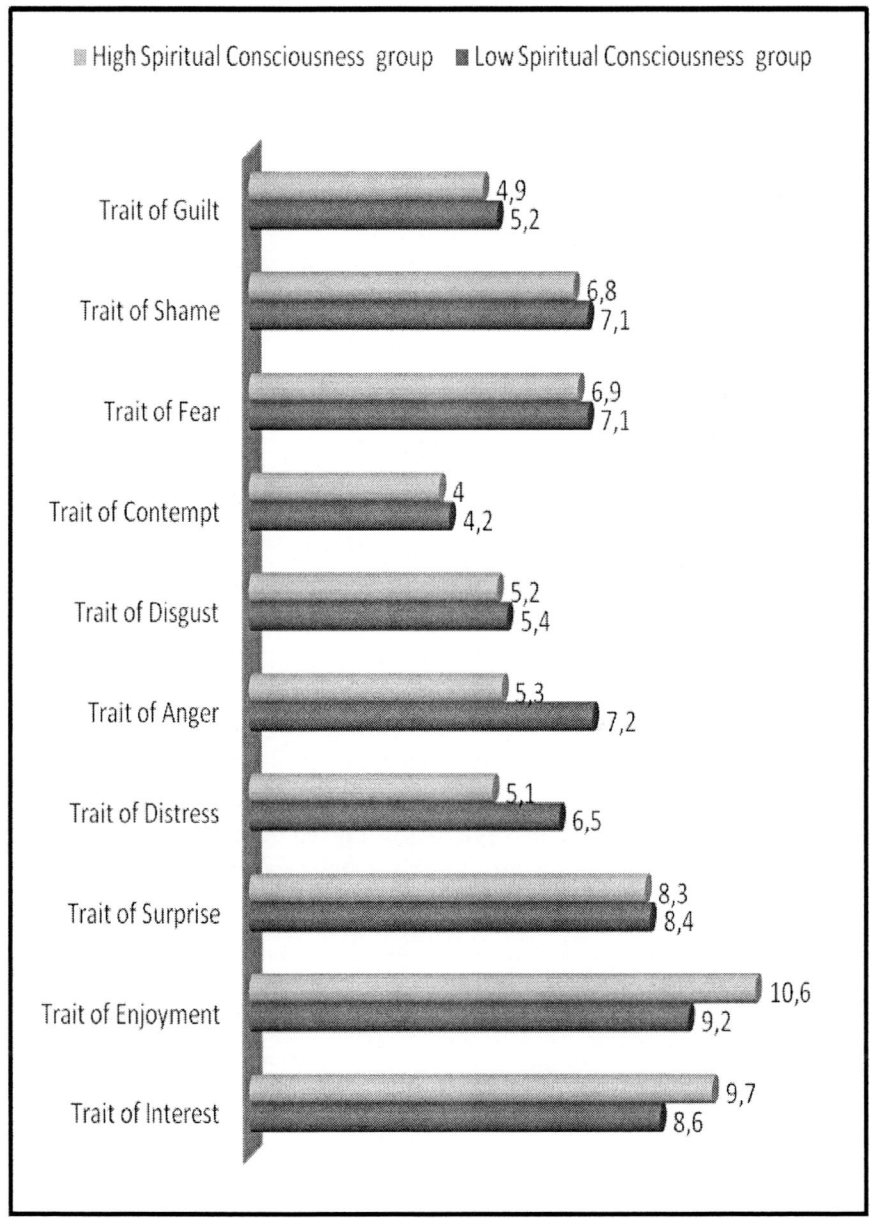

Figure 15. Descriptive statistics (mean value) of the results of emotions of Differentional Emotions Scale, employed in the groups arranged according to the New Spiritual Consciousness Scale.

Individuals with a higher spiritual consciousness were found to be willing to express the following emotions to a much larger extent than people with a lower spiritual consciousness:

> Trait of Interest (t=2,258, p<0,028)
> Trait of Enjoyment (t=3,231, p<0,002)

Individuals with a lower spiritual consciousness were found to be willing to express the following emotions to a much larger extent than people with a higher spiritual consciousness:

> Trait of Distress (t=2,915, p<0,005)
> Trait of Anger (t=3,544, p<0,001)

In terms of other emotions there was no significant difference between the two groups.

In the following part of the survey, we carried out a linear regression analysis (stepwise method) for the whole of the sample and for each gender separately to analyse the various sub-scales of Differentional Emotions Scale.

In the examination, the results achieved on the New Spiritual Consciousness Scale were the dependent variables and the various sub-scales of Differentional Emotions were the predictors (Chart 23).

Chart 24. The regression of the results scored on the New Spiritual Consciousness Scale on the various sub-scales measuring Differentional Emotions
(approved models; p<0,05)

Predictor	Béta	t	p<
Total: $F_{totál}=11,680$; $df=1/484$; $p<0,000$			
Trait of Anger	-0,380	-4,085	0,000
Trait of Interest	0,208	2,239	0,028
Women: $F_{totál}= 7,426$; $df=1/302$; $p<0,008$			
Trait of Anger	-0,287	-2,650	0,010
Trait of Interest	0,243	2,245	0,028
Men: $F_{totál}= 10,258$; $df=1/182$; $p<0,001$			
Trait of Anger	-0,398	4,597	0,000
Trait of Interest	0,216	2,028	0,036

At the entire sample, New Spiritual Consciousness showed a significant, close, positive relationship with the willingness to express Interest, and a significant, close, negative correlation with the expression of Anger, the two explaining 20,1% of the variance of New Spiritual Consciousness.

At the two genders, the tendency was the same as that observed at the entire sample. In the case of the women it explained 17,9% of the variance of New Spiritual Consciousness, whereas the figure was 21,2% in the case of the men.

It means that there is a direct proportion between the increase New Spiritual Consciousness and the increase of the willingness to express Interest/decrease of the willingness to express Anger at both sexes.

In the examination, the results achieved on the "Ego-dyastole" Subscale were the dependent variables and the various sub-scales of Differentional Emotions were the predictors (Chart 24).

Chart 24. The regression of the results scored on the Ego-dyastole" Subscale on the various sub-scales measuring Differentional Emotions (approved models; p<0,05

Predictor	Béta	t	p<
Total: $F_{totál}=15,151$; $df=1/484$; $p<0,001$			
Trait of Disgust	-0,301	-2,998	0,001
Trait of Contempt	-0,283	-2,825	0,006
Women: $F_{totál}=21,327$; $df=1/302$; $p<0,000$			
Trait of Contempt	-0,431	-4,398	0,000
Trait of Disgust	-0,346	-3,500	0,001
Men: $F_{totál}=14,144$; $df=1/182$; $p<0,002$			
Trait of Disgust	-0,298	-3,012	0,001
Trait of Contempt	-0,256	-2,652	0,017

In the whole sample, Ego-dyastole was found to be in a significant, close negative correlation with the willingness to express Disgust and Contempt, these two explaining 28,3% of the variance of Ego-dyastole.

At the two genders, the tendency was the same as that observed at the entire sample. In the case of the women it explained 36,9% of the variance of Ego-dyastole, whereas the figure was 23,8% in the case of the men.

It means that there is a direct proportion between the decline of the functions of the Ego and the decline of the willingness to express Disgust and Contempt at both sexes.

Chart 25. The regression of the results scored on the Alert consciousness in the present" Subscale on the various sub-scales measuring Differential Emotions (approved models; p<0,05)

Predictor	Béta	t	p<
Total: $F_{total}=5,290$; $df=1/484$; $p<0,024$			
Trait of Enjoyment	0,231	2,300	0,024
Women: $F_{total}=6,354$; $df=1/302$; $p<0,019$			
Trait of Enjoyment	0,254	2,451	0,019
Men: $F_{total}=5,214$; $df=1/182$; $p<0,028$			
Trait of Enjoyment	0,224	2,189	0,028

In the examination, the results achieved on the "Alert consciousness in the present" Subscale were the dependent variables and the various sub-scales of Differential Emotions were the predictors (Chart 25).

At the entire sample, Alert consciousness in the present was in a significant, close, positive interrelation with the inclination to express Enjoyment, which was responsible for a mere 5,3% of the variance of Alert consciousness in the present

At the two genders, the tendency was the same as that observed at the entire sample. In the case of the women it explained 6,2% of the variance of Alert consciousness in the present, whereas the figure was 4,9% in the case of the men.

It indicates that with the increase of alert consciousness in the present increases the willingness to express enjoyment. The tendency is the same at both sexes.

In the examination, the results achieved on the "Transcending the functions of Ego" Subscale were the dependent variables and the various sub-scales of Differential Emotions were the predictors (Chart 26).

At the entire sample, Transcending the functions of Ego was in a significant, close, positive interrelation with the inclination to express Interest, which was responsible for a mere 19,3% of the variance of Transcending the functions of Ego.

At the two genders, the tendency was the same as that observed at the entire sample. In the case of the women it explained 23,5% of the variance of Transcending the functions of Ego, whereas the figure was 16,9% in the case of the men.

Chart 26. The regression of the results scored on the Transcending the functions of Ego" Subscale on the various sub-scales measuring Differentional Emotions
(approved models; p<0,05)

Predictor	Béta	t	p<
Total: $F_{totál}=14,381$; $df=1/484$; $p<0,000$			
Trait of Interest	0,364	3,792	0,000
Women: $F_{totál}=22,731$; $df=1/302$; $p<0,000$			
Trait of Interest	0,485	4,768	0,000
Men: $F_{totál}=12,187$; $df=1/182$; $p<0,000$			
Trait of Interest	0,341	3,418	0,000

It indicates that with the increase of transcending the functions of Ego increases the willingness to express interest. The tendency is the same at both sexes.

8.1. DISCUSSION

We examined the connections between New Spiritual Consciousness and its specific components and the inclination to express various emotions.

It means that there is a direct proportion between the increase New Spiritual Consciousness and the increase of the willingness to express Interest/decrease of the willingness to express Anger at both sexes.

Our results indicate that New Spiritual Consciousness is in a close correlation with the inclination to express Interest and Anger. The tendency was found to be the same at both sexes.

Out of the specific dimensions of New Spiritual Consciousness, Ego-dyastole was found to be in a close connection with the willingness to express Disgust and Contempt, whereas Alert consciousness in the present showed a correlation with the inclination to express Enjoyment. It means that in parallel with the decline of the function of the Ego the inclination to express Disgust and Contempt also declines at both men and women. Similarly, in parallel with the increase of the alert consciousness in the present the inclination to express Enjoyment increases at both genders.

Chapter 9

PAIN BODY AND THE ANGER EXPRESSION

9.1. PAIN BODY EXPRESSION AND THE ANGER EXPRESSION

For the composition of the examination groups, the results scored on the Pain Body Expression Scale.

Students were arranged according to their position of the Pain Body Expression Scale. Students low on the Pain Body Expression Scale were in the first quarter (powerless Pain Body), whereas those who were high on the scale were put in the fourth quarter (powerful Pain Body).

Figure 16 contains the descriptive statistics (mean value) of the results of Anger Expression Scale, employed in the groups arranged according to the Pain Body Expression Scale.

The figure suggests that there is no considerable difference between the two groups in terms of Anger Expression.

The inclination to express Anger openly-Anger out-as a permanent characteristic feature was found to be considerably more common among individuals with a powerful Pain Body than among those with a powerless Pain Body (t=3,744, p<0,000). They experience the emotion of Anger more often, and they are ready to openly express their emotions to other people.

The inclination to suppress Anger-Anger in-as a permanent characteristic feature was found to be considerably more common among individuals with a powerless Pain Body than among those with a powerful Pain Body (t=3,505, p<0,000). They either suppress or control the emotion of Anger more often, and they are unwilling to openly express their emotions to other people.

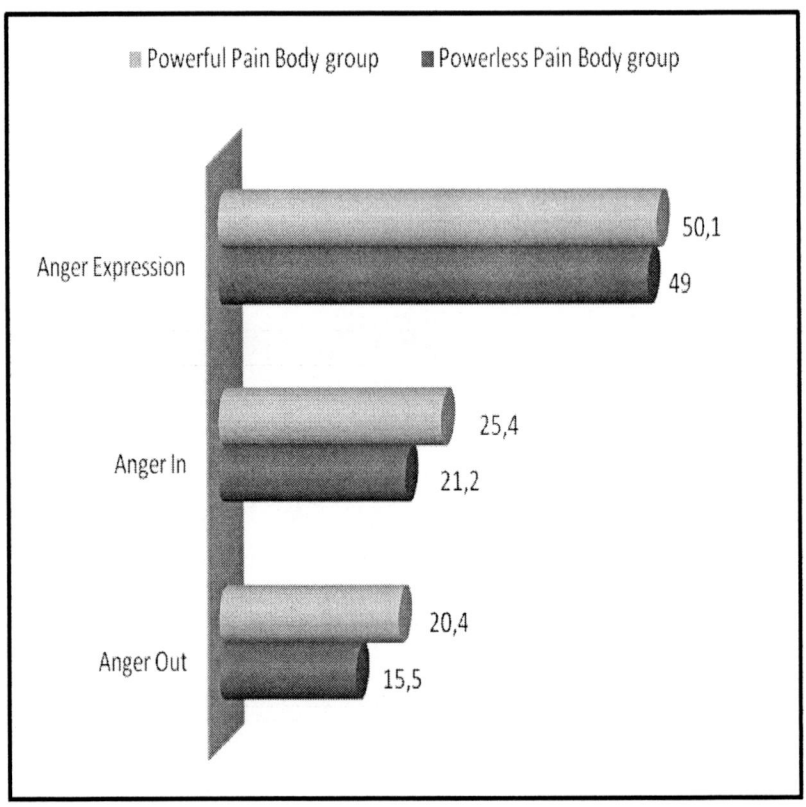

Figure 16. Descriptive statistics (mean value) of the results of Anger Expression Scale, employed in the groups arranged according to the Pain Body Expression Scale.

In the following part of the survey, we carried out a linear regression analysis (stepwise method) for the whole of the sample and for each gender separately to analyse the various sub-scales of Anger Expression Scale.

In the examination, the results achieved on the Pain Body Expression Scale were the dependent variables and the various sub-scales of Anger Expression Scale were the predictors (Chart 27).

At the entire sample, Pain Body was in a significant, close positive correlation with Anger out, and in a significant, close, negative correlation with Anger in, the two explaining 27,8% of the variance of Pain Body.

An examination of the two genders separately revealed that the tendency was the same in the case of both sexes, explaining 25,5% of the variance of the Pain Body in the case of the women and 28,2% in the case of the men.

Chart 27. The regression of the results scored on the Pain Body Expression Scale on the various sub-scales measuring Anger Expression Scale (approved models; p<0,05)

Predictor	Béta	t	p<
Total: $F_{totál}=17,919;\ df=1/484;\ p<0,000$			
Anger out	0,433	5,017	0,000
Anger in	-0,312	-3,533	0,001
Women: $F_{totál}=12,469;\ df=1/302;\ p<0,000$			
Anger out	0,442	4,971	0,000
Anger in	-0,269	-2,660	0,010
Men: $F_{totál}=17,658;\ df=1/182;\ p<0,000$			
Anger out	0,458	5,895	0,000
Anger in	-0,368	-3,981	0,000

It means that there is a direct proportion between the increase of the power of PB and the increase of the willingness to express Anger/decrease of the possibility to control or suppress Anger.

In the examination, the results achieved on the Exasperation" Subscale were the dependent variables and the various sub-scales of Anger Expression Scale were the predictors (Chart 28).

Chart 28. The regression of the results scored on the "Exasperation" Subscale on the various sub-scales measuring Anger Expression Scale (approved models; p<0,05)

Predictor	Béta	t	p<
Total: $F_{totál}=39,561;\ df=1/484;\ p<0,000$			
Anger out	0,544	6,290	0,000
Women: $F_{totál}=32,941;\ df=1/302;\ p<0,000$			
Anger out	0,555	5,739	0,000
Men: $F_{totál}=34,689;\ df=1/182;\ p<0,000$			
Anger out	0,512	5,184	0,000

At the whole group, Exasperation was found to be in a significant, close positive correlation with Anger out, which was responsible for 29,6% of the variance of Exasperation.

An examination of the two genders separately revealed that the tendency was the same in the case of both sexes, explaining 30,8% of the variance of the Pain Body in the case of the women and 28,7% in the case of the men.

It means that with the increase of Exasperation, the individual's willingness to openly express their Anger also increases.

In the examination, the results achieved on the "Grudge" Subscale were the dependent variables and the various sub-scales of Anger Expression Scale were the predictors (Chart 29).

At the entire sample, Grudge showed a significant, close negative correlation with only one dimension of Anger Expression, and that was Anger in. It was responsible for 11,6% of the variance of Grudge.

Chart 29. The regression of the results scored on the Grudge" Subscale on the various sub-scales measuring Anger Expression Scale (approved models; p<0,05)

Predictor	Béta	t	p<
Total: $F_{totál}=12,293$; $df=1/484$; $p<0,001$			
Anger in	-0,340	-3,506	0,001
Women: $F_{totál}=7,566$; $df=1/302$; $p<0,007$			
Anger in	-0,305	-2,751	0,007
Men: $F_{totál}=10,459$; $df=1/182$; $p<0,000$			
Anger in	-0,398	-3,951	0,000

Chart 30. The regression of the results scored on the Inflamability" Subscale on the various sub-scales measuring Anger Expression Scale (approved models; p<0,05)

Predictor	Béta	t	p<
Total: $F_{totál}=11,805$; $df=1/484$; $p<0,000$			
Anger in	-0,322	-3,578	0,000
Anger out	0,322	3,477	0,001
Women: $F_{totál}=8,334$; $df=1/302$; $p<0,001$			
Anger in	-0,324	-3,257	0,002
Anger out	0,280	2,644	0,010
Men: $F_{totál}=12,531$; $df=1/182$; $p<0,000$			
Anger in	-0,355	-3,753	0,000
Anger out	0,321	3,246	0,001

An examination of the two genders separately revealed that the tendency was the same in the case of both sexes, explaining 9,3% of the variance of the Pain Body in the case of the women and 12,4% in the case of the men.

It indicates that with the increase of Grudge, the individual's inclination to suppress the emotion of Anger declines.

In the examination, the results achieved on the "Inflammability" Subscale were the dependent variables and the various sub-scales of Anger Expression Scale were the predictors (Chart 30).

9.2. PAIN BODY CONTROL AND THE ANGER EXPRESSION

For the composition of the examination groups, the results scored on the Pain Body Control Scale.

Students were arranged according to their position of the Pain Body Control Scale. Students low on the Pain Body Control Scale were in the first quarter (powerless Control), whereas those who were high on the scale were put in the fourth quarter (powerful Control).

Figure 17 contains the descriptive statistics (mean value) of the results of Anger Expression Scale, employed in the groups arranged according to the Pain Body Control Scale.

The chart suggests that Anger Expression is more common among people with a powerless emotional control than among those with a powerful emotional control ($t=3,876$, $p<0,000$).

The inclination to express Anger openly (Anger out) as a permanent characteristic feature is significantly more common among individuals with a powerless emotional control than among those with a powerful emotional control ($t=4,257$, $p<0,000$). They experience the emotion of Anger a lot more often, and they are ready to openly express their emotions to other people.

In terms of the suppression of Anger (Anger in) as a permanent trait we detected no considerable difference between the two groups.

In the following part of the survey, we carried out a linear regression analysis (stepwise method) for the whole of the sample and for each gender separately to analyse the various sub-scales of Anger Expression Scale.

In the examination, the results achieved on the Pain Body Control Scale were the dependent variables and the various sub-scales of Anger Expression Scale were the predictors (Chart 31).

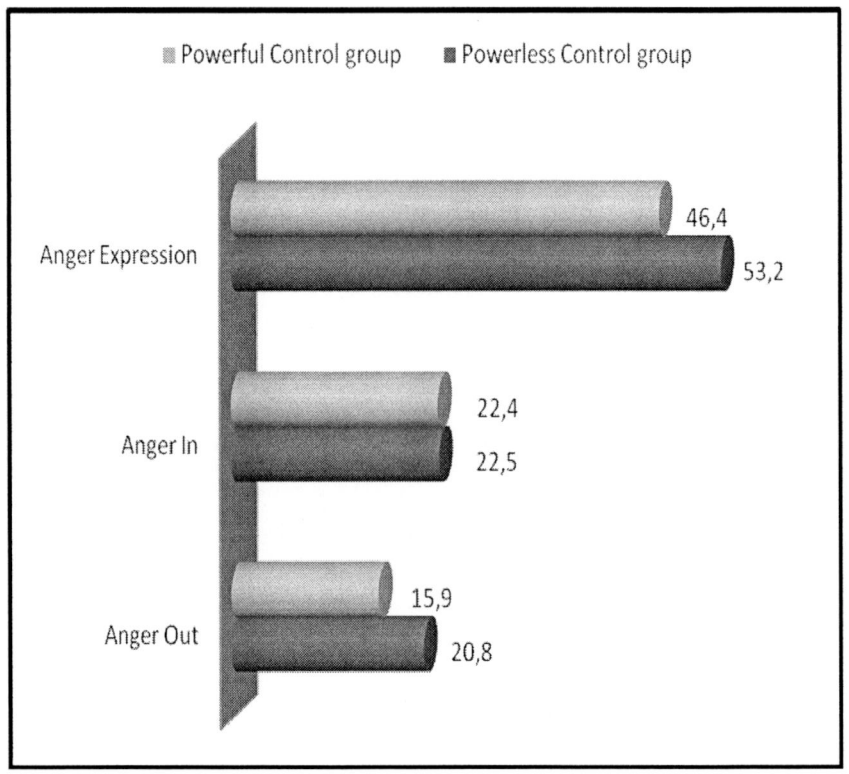

Figure 17. Descriptive statistics (mean value) of the results of Anger Expression Scale, employed in the groups arranged according to the Pain Body Control Scale.

Chart 31. The regression of the results scored on the Pain Body Control Scale on the various sub-scales measuring Anger Expression Scale (approved models; p<0,05)

Predictor	Béta	t	p<
Total: Ftotál=4,041; df=1/484; p<0,047			
Anger out	-0,203	-2,010	0,0047
Women: Ftotál= 4,598; df=1/302; p<0,039			
Anger out	-0,224	-2,542	0,039
Men: Ftotál= 4,125; df=1/182; p<0,045			
Anger out	-0,212	-2,125	0,045

At the entire sample, Pain Body was in a significant, close positive correlation with Anger out, and in a significant, close, negative correlation with Anger in, the two explaining 27,8% of the variance of Pain Body.

An examination of the two genders separately revealed that the tendency was the same in the case of both sexes, explaining 3,8% of the variance of the Pain Body in the case of the women and 5,2% in the case of the men.

It means that there is a direct proportion between the increase of the power of Pain Body and the increase of the willingness to express Anger/decrease of the possibility to control or suppress Anger.

9.3. Discussion

We examined the connections between Pain Body/Pain Body Control and the expression of Anger.

Our research findings show a close correlation between Pain Body and all the two versions of Anger Expression at both genders.

It means that with the decline of the power of Pain Body the inclination of expressing Anger declines similarly and the individual's capacity to suppress or control Anger increases, and the other way around.

Out of the structural components of Pain Body, Exasperation was linked only to Anger out, Grudge to Anger in and Inflammability to both manifestations of Anger Expression. The tendency was found to be the same at both genders.

It means that with the decline of Exasperation, the individual's inclination to openly express the emotion of Anger, and with the decline of Grudge the individual's inclination to suppress or control Anger increases. In parallel with the decrease of Inflammability, the individual's inclination to express the emotion of Anger decreases similarly, and the person's capacity to suppress or control Anger increases.

An examination of the connection between Pain Body Control and Anger Expression revealed that emotional control was in connection only with Anger out, and not with the other manifestation of Anger Expression. It was the same at both sexes.

It means that there is a direct proportion between the increase of the power of Pain Body and the increase of the willingness to express Anger/decrease of the possibility to control or suppress Anger.

Chapter 10

NEW SPIRITUAL CONSCIOUSNESS AND THE ANGER EXPRESSION

For the composition of the examination groups, the results scored on the New Spiritual Consciousness Scale.

Students were arranged according to their position of the New Spiritual Consciousness Scale. Students low on the New Spiritual Consciousness Scale were in the first quarter, whereas those who were high on the scale were put in the fourth quarter.

Figure 18 contains the descriptive statistics (mean value) of the results of Anger Expression Scale, employed in the groups arranged according to the New Spiritual Consciousness Scale.

The figure suggests that there is no considerable difference between people with lower and higher new spiritual consciousness in terms of the ways of expressing Anger.

In the following part of the survey, we carried out a linear regression analysis (stepwise method) for the whole of the sample and for each gender separately to analyse the various sub-scales of Anger Expression Scale.

In the examination, the results achieved on the New Spiritual Consciousness Scale were the dependent variables and the various sub-scales of Anger Expression Scale were the predictors (Chart 32).

At the entire sample, New Spiritual Consciousness was in a significant, close negative correlation with Anger out, explaining only 4,7% of the variance of New Spiritual Consciousness.

An examination of the two genders separately revealed that the tendency was the same in the case of both sexes, explaining 6,2% of the variance of the Pain Body in the case of the women and 3,4% in the case of the men.

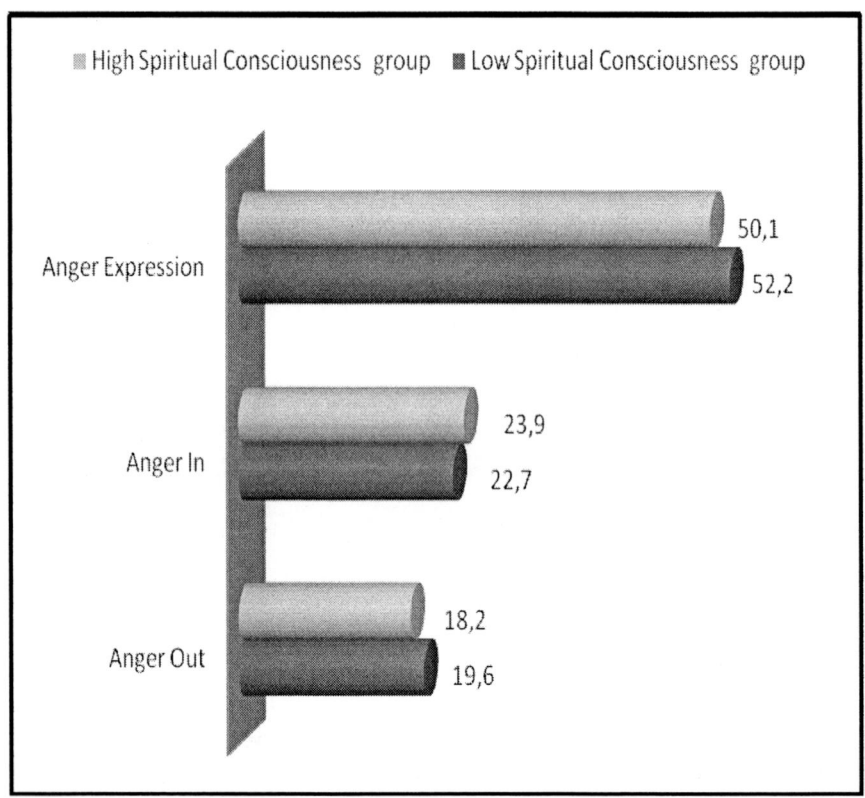

Figure 18. Descriptive statistics (mean value) of the results of Anger Expression Scale, employed in the groups arranged according to the New Spiritual Consciousness Scale.

Chart 32. The regression of the results scored on the New Spiritual Consciousness Scale on the various sub-scales measuring Anger Expression Scale (approved models; p<0,05)

Predictor	Béta	t	p<
Total: $F_{totál}=4,685$; $df=1/484$; $p<0,033$			
Anger out	-0,218	-2,164	0,033
Women: $F_{totál}= 5,368$; $df=1/302$; $p<0,028$			
Anger out	-0,234	-2,341	0,028
Men: $F_{totál}= 4,254$; $df=1/182$; $p<0,037$			
Anger out	-0,207	-2,002	0,037

Chart 33. The regression of the results scored on the Ego-dyastole" Subscale on the various sub-scales measuring Anger Expression Scale (approved models; p<0,05)

Predictor	Béta	t	p<
Total: $F_{totál}=18,812$; $df=1/484$; $p<0,000$			
Anger out	-0,402	-4,402	0,000
Anger in	0,379	4,320	0,000
Women: $F_{totál}=15,801$; $df=1/302$; $p<0,000$			
Anger out	-0,438	-4,414	0,000
Anger in	0,328	3,303	0,001
Men: $F_{totál}=16,458$; $df=1/182$; $p<0,000$			
Anger out	-0,392	-4,412	0,000
Anger in	0,336	3,412	0,001

It indicates that there is a reverse proportion between the increase of new spiritual consciousness and the urge to express Anger openly.

In the examination, the results achieved on the "Ego-dyastole" Subscale were the dependent variables and the various sub-scales of Anger Expression Scale were the predictors (Chart 33).

At the entire sample, Ego-dyastole was in a significant, close negative correlation with Anger out, and in significant, close positive correlation with Anger in out of the dimensions of Ego-dyastole, all these explaining 28,8% of the variance of Ego-dyastole.

An examination of the two genders separately revealed that the tendency was the same in the case of both sexes, explaining 28,3% of the variance of the Pain Body in the case of the women and 29,4% in the case of the men.

It suggests that there is a direct proportion between the decline of the functions of the Ego and the increase of the urge to suppress Anger, and thus the possibility of the open expression of Anger also decreases.

In the examination, the results achieved on the "Alert consciousness in the present" Subscale were the dependent variables and the various sub-scales of Anger Expression Scale were the predictors (Chart 34).

At the entire sample, Alert consciousness in the present was in a significant, close negative correlation with Anger in, explaining a mere 7,9% of the variance of Alert consciousness in the present.

An examination of the two genders separately revealed that the tendency was the same in the case of both sexes, explaining 9,2% of the variance of the Pain Body in the case of the women and 6,4% in the case of the men.

Chart 34. The regression of the results scored on the Alert consciousness in the present" Subscale on the various sub-scales measuring Anger Expression Scale
(approved models; p<0,05)

Predictor	Béta	t	p<
Total: $F_{totál}=8,009$; $df=1/484$; $p<0,006$			
Anger in	-0,280	-2,830	0,006
Women: $F_{totál}=7,548$; $df=1/302$; $p<0,010$			
Anger in	-0,268	-2,236	0,010
Men: $F_{totál}=9,258$; $df=1/182$; $p<0,004$			
Anger in	-0,301	-3,121	0,004

It suggests that there is a direct proportion between the increase of the alert consciousness in the present and the decrease of the willingness to suppress Anger.

In the course of our research, were not able to detect any considerable interrelation between Transcending the functions of Ego and the willingness to express various emotions.

10.1. DISCUSSION

In the course of our research project we wished to survey the connections of New Spiritual Consciousness and its specific components and the ways of expressing the emotion of Anger.

Our results indicate that Anger out was the only dimension of Anger Expression that showed a close correlation with New Spiritual Consciousness. It was the same at both genders. It means that there is a direct proportion between the increase of the new spiritual consciousness and the decrease of the individual's inclination to openly express Anger. It appears to be the same at both genders.

Ego-dyastole was the dimension of New Spiritual Consciousness that was found to be in a close connection with both manifestations of Anger Expression.

It suggests that there is a direct proportion between the decline of the functions of the Ego and the increase of the urge to suppress Anger, and thus the possibility of the open expression of Anger also decreases

Anger in was the dimension of Anger Expression that was in a close connection with Alert consciousness in the present.

It suggests that there is a direct proportion between the increase of the alert consciousness in the present and the decrease of the willingness to suppress Anger.

In the course of our research, were not able to detect any considerable interrelation between Transcending the functions of Ego and the willingness to express various emotions.

Chapter 11

PAIN BODY EXPRESSION SCALE

Please, read all statements carefully and mark the alternative that best describes your emotions and behavior by the number of each statement on the answer sheet, according to the following criteria:

**Scale. 1= virtually never, 2=sometimes, 3= frequently, 4=almost always
Before submitting the sheet, please check whether you have answered all the statements**

1. I become upset without any particular reason	1	2	3	4
2. I harbour resentment against others	1	2	3	4
3. I easily become angry	1	2	3	4
4. I feel remorse	1	2	3	4
5. My moods change rapidly	1	2	3	4
6. I become depressed or sad without any particular reason	1	2	3	4
7. People make me nervous	1	2	3	4
8. I am overcome by self-pity	1	2	3	4
9. I am often overcome by my emotions	1	2	3	4
10. I have negative ideas about myself	1	2	3	4
11. I am envious of others	1	2	3	4
12. I easily offend others	1	2	3	4
13. Small, insignificant things trigger intensive emotions in me	1	2	3	4
14. I easily criticize others	1	2	3	4
15. I am often overcome by my emotions unexpectedly	1	2	3	4
16. I am unhappy	1	2	3	4
17. I am impatient with others	1	2	3	4

Please give your age, gender, and occupation.

Age..

Gender... ....

Occupation...

Chapter 12

USE OF THE PAIN BODY EXPRESSION SCALE

COMPLETING THE QUESTIONNAIRE AND THE PROCESS OF ASSESSMENT

The questionnaire for self-description may be used for individual and group surveys as well.

In order to provide the respondents with appropriate circumstances for completing the questionnaire, it is advisable to choose a noise-free and well-lit room.

If a respondent has difficulties in reading the questionnaire (dyslexia), the person conducting the survey may read out the questions loud, and note down the answers of the respondent

Instructions on the Questionnaire

Please, read all statements carefully and mark the alternative that best describes your emotions and behavior by the number of each statement on the answer sheet, according to the following criteria:

Scale: 1= virtually never, 2=sometimes, 3= frequently, 4=almost always

Before submitting the sheet, please check whether you have answered all the statements.

Our preliminary experience suggests that the average college student will need approximately ten to ten minutes to complete the questionnaire.

The first step in the manual assessment of the questionnaire is summing up the points given to the items that make up the dimensions.

The items belonging to the specific dimensions are shown in Chart 35.

Chart 35. The items that belong to the specific dimensions of the Pain Body Expression Scale

Sub-scale of the Pain Body Expression Scale	Items
"Exasperation" sub-scale	1, 3, 5, 7, 12, 14, 17
" Grudge" sub-scale	2, 4, 10, 11, 16
" Inflammability" sub-scale	6, 8, 9, 13, 15

It is possible to well use the questionnaire for research.

Chapter 13

PAIN BODY CONTROL SCALE

Please, read all statements carefully and mark the alternative that best describes your emotions and behavior by the number of each statement on the answer sheet, according to the following criteria:

**Scale. 1= virtually never, 2=sometimes, 3= frequently, 4=almost always
Before submitting the sheet, please check whether
you have answered all the statements**

1. I am able to control my emotions	1	2	3	4
2. I am able to forget about old offenses	1	2	3	4
3. When I realize that an emotions overcomes me, I am able to consciously suppress it	1	2	3	4
4. I am able to contemplate my emotions like an outsider	1	2	3	4
5. I do not identify with my emotions, I simply allow them to happen	1	2	3	4
6. When I am suffering emotionally, I do not escape, I make efforts to consciously face the emotion concerned	1	2	3	4
7. I am able to focus my attention on the present, instead of re-living old emotions	1	2	3	4

Please give your age, gender, and occupation

Age..

Gender..

Occupation..

Chapter 14

USE OF THE PAIN BODY CONTROL SCALE

COMPLETING THE QUESTIONNAIRE AND THE PROCESS OF ASSESSMENT

The questionnaire for self-description may be used for individual and group surveys as well.

In order to provide the respondents with appropriate circumstances for completing the questionnaire, it is advisable to choose a noise-free and well-lit room.

If a respondent has difficulties in reading the questionnaire (dyslexia), the person conducting the survey may read out the questions loud, and note down the answers of the respondent

Instructions on the Questionnaire

Please, read all statements carefully and mark the alternative that best describes your emotions and behavior by the number of each statement on the answer sheet, according to the following criteria:

Scale. 1= virtually never, 2=sometimes, 3= frequently, 4=almost always

Before submitting the sheet, please check whether you have answered all the statements.

Our preliminary experience suggests that the average college student will need approximately ten to ten minutes to complete the questionnaire.

In the manual assessment of the questionnaire is summing up the points given to the items that make up the dimensions.

It is possible to well use the questionnaire for research.

REFERENCES

[1] Tolle, E. (1997): *The Power of Now.* New Wordl Library, Novato.
[2] Tolle, E. (2006): *Új föld [New Earth].* Agykontroll Kft., Budapest.
[3] Kleinginna, P.R., and Kleinginna, A.M. (1981): A categorized list of emotion definitions with suggestions for a consensual definition. *Motivation and Emotion.* 5: 345-379.
[4] Fischer, K., and Shaver, P.R., and Carnochran, P. (1990): How emotions develop and how they organize development. Cognition and Emotion, 4: 81-127.
[5] Urbán, R. (2004): Érzelmek. [Emotions] In: N. Kollár K–Szabó É. (Szerk.): *Pszichológia pedagógusoknak.* Osiris Kiadó, Budapest, 95-118.
[6] Cole, M., and Cole S. R. (1997): *Fejlődéslélektan [Development Psychology].* Osiris Kiadó, Budapest
[7] Izard, C.E. (1971): *The Face of Emotions.* Appleton-Century-Crofts, New York.
[8] Izard, C.E. (1991): *The Psychology of Emotions.* Plenum Press, New York.
[9] Oláh, A. (2005): *Érzelmek, megküzdés és optimális élmény.* Trefor Kiadó, Budapest.
[10] Mayer, J.D., and Salovey, P. (1993): The intelligence of emotional intelligence. *Intelligence*, 17: 433-442.
[11] Bar-On, R. (1997): *Bar-On Emotional Quotient Inventory: technical manual.* Toronto, ON: Multi-Health Systems.
[12] Goleman, D. (1995): *Emotional intelligence.* Bantam Books, New York.
[13] Forgas, J. P. (2001): Affektív intelligencia: az érzések hatása a társas gondolkodásra és viselkedésre. [Affective Intelligence: The Role of

Affect in Social Thinking and Behavior] In: Ciarrochi, J., and Forgas, J.P., and Mayer, J.D. (szerk.) *Az érzelmi intelligencia a mindennapi életben [Emotional Intelligence in Everyday Life]*. Kairosz Kiadó, Budapest, 77-100.

[14] Taylor, G.J. (2001):Alacsony érzelmi intelligenciaszint és lelki betegség. [Low Emotional Intelligence and Mental Illness] In: Ciarrochi, J., and Forgas, J.P., and Mayer, J.D. (szerk.) *Az érzelmi intelligencia a mindennapi életben. [Emotional Intelligence in Everyday Life]*.Kairosz Kiadó, Budapest, 103-122.

[15] Bar-On, R. (2001): Érzelmi intelligencia és önmegvalósítás. [Emotional Intelligence and Self-Actualization]. In: Ciarrochi, J., and Forgas, J.P., and Mayer, J.D. (szerk.) *Az érzelmi intelligencia a mindennapi életben. [Emotional Intelligence in Everyday Life]*.Kairosz Kiadó, Budapest, 123-141.

[16] Fitness, J. (2001): Érzelmi intelligencia és házasság. In: Ciarrochi, J., and Forgas, J.P., and Mayer, J.D. (szerk.) *Az érzelmi intelligencia a mindennapi életben. [Emotional Intelligence in Everyday Life]*.Kairosz Kiadó, Budapest, 143-161.

[17] Flury, J., and Ickes, W. (2001): Érzelmi intelligencia és empátiás pontosság. In: Ciarrochi, J., and Forgas, J.P., and Mayer, J.D. (szerk.) *Az érzelmi intelligencia a mindennapi életben. [Emotional Intelligence in Everyday Life]*.Kairosz Kiadó, Budapest, 163-186.

[18] Elias, M.J., and Hunter, L., and Kress, J.S. (2001): Érzelmi intelligencia és nevelés. In: Ciarrochi, J., and Forgas, J.P., and Mayer, J.D. (szerk.) *Az érzelmi intelligencia a mindennapi életben. [Emotional Intelligence in Everyday Life]*.Kairosz Kiadó, Budapest, 187-208.

[19] Mayer, J.D., and DiPaolo, M.T., and Salovey, P. (1990): Perceiving affective content in ambiguous visual stimuli: A component of emotional intelligence. *Journal of Personality Assesment*, 54: 772-781.

[20] Mayer, J.D., and Salovey, P., and Caruso, D.R. (1999): Emotional intelligence meets traditional standards for an intelligence. *Intelligence*, 27: 267-298.

[21] Bar-On, R. (2006): The Bar-On model of emotional-social intelligence (ESI). *Psicothema*, 18: 13-25.

[22] Margitics, F. (2009): New Spiritual Consciousness: Theory and Research. Nova Publishers, New York.

[23] Spielberger, C.D., and Johnson, E.H., and Russel, S.F., and Crane, R.J., and Jacobs, G.A., and Worden, T.J. (1985): The experience and expression of anger: Construction and validation of an Anger Expression Scale. In: Chesney, M.A., and Rosenman, R.H. (Eds): *Anger and hostility in cardiovascular and behavioral disorders.* Hemisphere/McGraw-Hill, New York.

INDEX

A

adaptation, 21
aggression, 21
alertness, 41, 42
alters, 42
anger, viii, 21, 87
assessment, 1, 5, 80, 84
assimilation, 5
avoidance, 3

B

behavioral disorders, 87
breakdown, 23, 24

C

central nervous system, 2
childhood, vii, 7, 8
cognitive process, 2
collective unconscious, 8
college students, 10, 17, 19
compilation, 9, 15
complexity, 5
composition, 23, 29, 36, 43, 49, 55, 63, 67, 71
comprehension, 5
consciousness, viii, 31, 39, 41, 42, 55, 56, 58, 60, 61, 71, 73, 74, 75
consent, 19
correlation, 9, 10, 15, 16, 25, 26, 30, 33, 34, 35, 41, 46, 47, 48, 49, 53, 59, 61, 64, 66, 69, 71, 73, 74
correlations, 9, 10, 15, 16
creative process, 3
creativity, 2
criticism, 12
cultural differences, 4
culture, 2

D

decay, 3
dependent variable, 33, 34, 35, 41, 46, 48, 51, 58, 59, 60, 64, 65, 66, 67, 71, 73
depression, vii, 7
deviation, 19
dispersion, 9, 15
dyslexia, 79, 83

E

emotion, vii, 1, 2, 3, 7, 16, 17, 21, 46, 47, 63, 64, 67, 69, 74, 81, 85
emotional information, 5
emotional intelligence, 4, 5, 6, 7, 85, 86
emotional reactions, vii, 7
emotional state, 3
ESI, 86
examinations, 4
experiences, 21
exploration, 5

external environment, 5

F

facial expression, 2
facilitators, 6
factor analysis, 10, 12, 17
feelings, 1, 5, 6
foundations, vii, 8

G

guidance, 7
guilt, 13, 26

H

hostility, 87
Hunter, 86

I

impulses, 6
independence, 7
Independence, 7
information processing, 5
intelligence, 4, 5, 6, 7, 8, 34, 85, 86
interference, 3
internal consistency, 9, 15
interpersonal relations, 6
interpersonal relationships, 6
interrelations, 12, 17, 38, 42

L

learning, 2, 4

M

majority, 20
management, 5
marriage, 5
median, 19
memory, 2
mental processes, 8
motivation, 2, 5, 6

N

negative emotions, vii, 7, 8
negative relation, 35
nervous system, 2, 3
nervousness, 12, 26
noise, 79, 83

O

one dimension, 66
opportunities, 4

P

pain, vii, 7, 8
parallel, 49, 61, 69
personal identity, 8
pleasure, 3, 7
positive correlation, 41, 46, 47, 48, 49, 64, 66, 69, 73
positive emotions, 6
positive relationship, 52, 59
project, viii, 26, 42, 74
psychology, 1

Q

quality of life, 5

R

reactions, vii, 1, 7, 42
reading, 79, 83
reality, 8
recognition, vii, 5
regression, 32, 34, 35, 36, 40, 41, 45, 46, 47, 48, 50, 52, 58, 59, 60, 61, 64, 65, 66, 67, 68, 71, 72, 73, 74
regression analysis, 32, 40, 45, 50, 58, 64, 67, 71
reliability, 9, 10, 11, 15, 16, 17, 21
resentment, 10, 11, 13, 77

S

self-actualization, 5

self-awareness, 7
self-confidence, 3
self-control, 7
self-esteem, 7
sex, 56
shame, 3
shyness, 3
social environment, 4
social group, 7
social relations, 2
social skills, 6
socialization, 4
spirituality, 41
standard deviation, 19
statistics, 23, 24, 25, 29, 30, 31, 32, 33, 37, 38, 39, 40, 43, 44, 45, 49, 50, 51, 55, 56, 57, 63, 64, 67, 68, 71, 72
suppression, 21, 67

surplus, 9, 10, 15, 16
survey, 32, 40, 41, 45, 50, 58, 64, 67, 71, 74, 79, 83

T

thoughts, vii, 7, 8, 42
traits, 43, 44

U

unhappiness, 13, 26

V

validation, 87
visual stimuli, 86